"Sensational! No counting calories. No difficult diet to follow. Jack simplifies the process of what, when, and how to eat and connects you with the importance of being consistent."

—Ian Baker Finch
Professional Golfer and 1991 British Open Champion

"Groppel's approach to nutrition in *The Anti-Diet Book* is scientifically based, yet presented in a very entertaining and practical way. His extensive work in the corporate and athletic arenas provides the experience to effectively inform those with the most demanding of schedules."

—Mike Nishihara, Director of Athletic Development
National Institute of Fitness and Sport

"Jack Groppel's program for utilizing and managing nutrition to optimize performance has added a new dimension to physicians' lives both personally and professionally."

—Nicholas de Bourgknecht, Director
CIBA Benelux, Europe

"*The Anti-Diet Book* is a clearly written, well researched work on an often touched but seldom understood subject with one glaring difference: It works! Groppel gives the reader insight into how nutrition affects our moods, energy levels, and overall health. Understanding these concepts is absolutely critical for anyone interested in performing at peak levels."

—Mike Richter, Goalie
New York Rangers Hockey Team

"*The Anti-Diet Book* shows why dieting does not work and why eating the right combination of foods six or seven times a day, plus drinking a sufficient amount of water and juices, benefits you mentally, physically, and nutritionally. This book is for everyone from the athlete to the businessperson, the housewife, the student, or the couch potato. Read it, absorb it, and live by it!"

—Dave Nelson, First Base Coach
Cleveland Indians Baseball Team

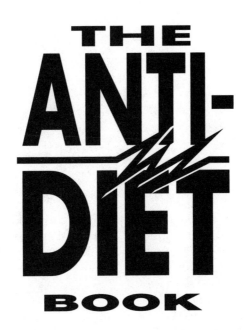

THE ANTI-DIET BOOK

Learn how to eat strategically,
perform on demand, and train
your metabolism to
burn fat more efficiently

Jack L. Groppel, Ph.D.

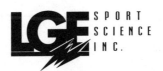

LGE SPORT SCIENCE INC.

LGE Sport Science, Inc.
9757 Lake Nona Rd.
Orlando, FL 32827
(407) 438-9911
fax (407) 438-6667

Second edition

Printed in the United States of America
10 9 8 7 6 5 4 3 2

ISBN 1-890009-04-0
Also available on audio cassette: ISBN 1-890009-05-9

Editorial/text design/production:
Executive Excellence
1344 East 1120 South
Provo, UT 84606
(801) 375-4060

Cover design by Chenoweth & Faulkner
Printed by Publishers Press

To Jan:
Thank you for your love,
friendship, and support.

ACKNOWLEDGMENTS

I am indebted to many people for their encouragement and support in conducting the research for this project and in completing this manuscript.

First, to my family: Jan, Dana, and Kirsten; my parents, Howard and Pauline Groppel; and my sister, Ruth Ann Kincaid, and her family. Without their love and support, this project would have been impossible. We have all grown through this study of nutrition and human performance.

To Dr. Jim Loehr: a better friend and colleague would be hard to find. And to Pat Etcheberry, who is a great friend as well as the best fitness trainer in sports today.

To the entire staff at LGE Sport Science, Inc., for their devotion to the cause we believe in. Special thanks goes to Becky Johnson, whose vision and dedication help to guide our company into the future.

To Warren and Kitty Jamison, without whose tireless work this manuscript would have been virtually impossible to complete.

To the two primary mentors in my life—Dr. Chuck Dillman and Dr. Bob Singer—who have helped me in the arduous path of understanding human performance.

To my colleagues and friends who are the rock of support and source of a plethora of ideas: Bill Wicks, Paul Roetert, Ron Woods, Tim and Tom Gullikson, Stan Smith, Vic Braden, and Bill Kraemer.

To Ken Shelton, Trent Price, and the entire staff at Executive Excellence for the fine editing involved in producing this book.

Special thanks goes to ESHA Research in Salem, Oregon (1-800-659-ESHA), the leading nutrition software producer, for the use of their tremendous software in analyzing the various programs and products found in this book.

CONTENTS

INTRODUCTION

"Food is an important part of a balanced diet."
—Fran Lebowitz

In the industrialized West, especially the United States, we are preoccupied with eating to a more pervasive extent than past civilizations. With us, business deals commonly get pushed forward during meals. Sporting events revolve around concessions and food. At resort hotels, organizing meals has developed into a meeting planner's most important function.

How Well Do You Fuel Your Ferrari?

You are a high-performance machine, a Ferrari, if you will. Consider this central question: How well do you fuel your Ferrari?

Imagine for a moment a big diesel truck driving up to your house and unloading a Ferrari you inherited from your late Uncle Ed. You're jumping up and down with eagerness to take the car for a spin, but its tank is empty. The only fuel available is the viscous diesel fuel in the eighteen-wheeler still idling in front of your house. Would you put the diesel fuel in your Ferrari or wait until you could get some high-octane gasoline? I'll wager you wouldn't risk wreaking havoc on the high-performance engine by clogging it with diesel fuel.

But do you exercise the same caution about how you fuel your other Ferrari, your body? After all, you could replace the Ferrari's automobile engine. Since replacing body parts is a severely limited option, shouldn't you exercise even greater care in how you fuel *it*? In place of the Ferrari engine's parts machined to close tolerances, your body has organs and arteries susceptible to clogging or other damage if improperly fueled. Your entire body consists of cells and tissues dependent on proper fuel for continued life, health, and high performance.

How well you fuel your Ferrari not only determines how well you perform, but fuel quality and quantity also have an enormous impact on how long your Ferrari (your body) will keep running. Unfortunately, these grim thoughts represent reality.

The Extraordinary Laboratory of Sports Nutrition

As everyone knows, sports demand great physical exertion and place extraordinary emotional pressure on professional athletes to perform at their highest level. Nowhere else are the differences between good and bad nutrition so quickly apparent, so easily observed, and so decisive. Working with thousands of outstanding sport and Corporate Athletes has given me a knowledge and understanding of nutrition I could have gained in no other way.

Corporate Athletes (businesspeople under pressure to perform at high levels for long periods) and sport athletes have similar needs for power-providing and health-building nutrition. In addition to my work with corporate executives over the past 20 years, I have also had the privilege of working with many world-class athletes who compete in many different sports—baseball, basketball, football, ice hockey, car racing, equestrian, figure skating, golf, gymnastics, swimming, tennis, racquetball, table tennis, and badminton.

Although these sports involve vastly different physical skills, the basic elements of discipline, fitness, mental toughness, and adequate recovery (nutrition, sleep, and relaxation), are vital to success in all of them. The same applies to success in business or any other field of human endeavor.

Set a World-Class Training Table

Today's athletic training table contains high complex carbohydrate foods like rice, pasta, potatoes and other vegetables, fruits, and whole grains, along with low-fat meats such as fish, turkey, and chicken. The goal is moderate to high carbohydrate intake and moderate protein consumption. Complex carbohydrates sustain the high-energy level that maximum performance requires, although it's also vital to meet your protein and fat requirements.

Studying the world's greatest athletes and examining their nutritional needs for top performance brings me to a very interesting conclusion: What works for them in competition is exactly what you need to perform at high levels cognitively and also to maintain optimum health. What the professional athlete in sports requires, you, as a Corporate Athlete in business, also require to sustain maximum performance over your long workdays, week after week, year after year.

The diet that helps a great athlete perform at a very high level is the same diet you should have to stay healthy and perform well in life. Again, it includes moderate to high amounts of complex carbohydrates from fruits, vegetables, and whole grains; moderate amounts of protein, largely from fish and grains but also from meat; and low amounts of fat—as much as possible of the unsaturated kind found in plants and fish. That's what I recommend you eat every day.

Some of the athletes I've worked with include:

Ian Baker-Finch . . . . .Golf
Wendy Bruce . . . . .Gymnastics
Jennifer Capriati .Tennis
Michael Chang . . . . .Tennis
Jim Courier . . . . .Tennis
Ken Daneyko . . . . .Ice Hockey
Mike Dunham . . . . .Ice Hockey
Kelly Leadbetter . . . . .Golf
Todd Martin . . . . .Tennis
Lisa Raymond . . . . .Tennis
Mike Richter . . . . .Ice Hockey
Chanda Rubin . . . . .Tennis
Arantxa Sánchez-Vicario . . . . .Tennis
Monica Seles . . . . .Tennis
Petr Sykora .Ice Hockey
Malivai Washington . . . . .Tennis
Nicole Wasilewski . . . . .Figure Skating

If your lifestyle involves effort and stress; if you have to make tough decisions when they count; if you go outdoors to pursue a hobby, an interest, or a duty; if you're a performer, whether mentally or physically; if you are called upon to organize and schedule, even if it's simply a car pool—you need to know about nutrition. In particular, businesspeople who work long hours and cope with world-class stress need world-class recovery in all its forms to sustain high performance.

Physically active people have far greater nutritional needs than dyed-in-the-wool couch potatoes who disdain eating and exercising sensibly until they have a heart attack or get some other urgent wake-up call.

In this book I will follow scientifically proven nutritional facts and principles rather than preferences. And I state those facts and principles in basic language so that anyone whose lifework is not nutrition, exercise, and general health building will understand easily. I'm presenting scientifically based material designed to be implemented immediately in your life.

The *New York Times* recently editorialized, "The world's increase in obesity continues despite a growing awareness that it's negative. . . . Figures on children show that obesity among the world's youth is increasing at an even faster rate than we're seeing in adults."

Much remains to be done, not only in America, but worldwide. Yet it all starts with each individual, who alone is responsible for his or her lifestyle.

Eat Anything You Want

When I meet a new family of sport hopefuls, my first sentence usually causes the parents to say, "What?" When I work with young athletes, I tell them, "I want you to know right now that you can eat anything you want!"

The kids shout, "Yes!" They turn to Mom and Dad and say, "I like this guy!" The parents panic. The reason I start that way is because about 15 years ago I gave a talk in Arizona to a group of great young tennis players, ages 12 and under. These young people could hit forehands at about 40 miles an hour.

We discussed nutrition. They had already competed in the morning, and they were going to compete again in the afternoon. I didn't impose any dietary regulations, but after hearing my talk the parents took their children out to lunch on salads, pasta, and whole-grain breads.

When everyone returned at 1:30, I was standing behind the tennis court speaking to the parents of a boy who was playing. He served the first game and lost his serve. They changed ends, and as he walked by the fence he told me, "If you hadn't made my mom feed me that stuff, I would have won that first game!"

He blamed losing the game totally on me. So I tell people I am not responsible for people winning or losing. What I'm going to do is give you the best information and research I know. Everything is documented in scientific journals and nutritional science. However, the decision to make the right choices and compete at the highest level is up to you.

Chapter 1

WHY ANTI-DIETING WORKS AND DIETING DOESN'T

"If you die before you're 130, you die of bad management."
—Peter Hansen

The American weight-loss industry rakes in nearly 50 billion dollars a year. It's an astonishing amount of money in view of one fact: Most of the people who actually lose weight gain every pound back after they go off their latest diet. Worse yet, this yo-yo process often puts on extra pounds.

The Diet Dilemma

You've heard it before—diets don't work! And you've also heard all the clichés about diet and weight-loss programs:
• The first three letters in diet are D - I - E.
• Diet is a four-letter word.
• Once you go on a diet, you must go off the diet.
• Dieting is a roller-coaster lifestyle.
Dieting exerts a strong appeal. Nearly everyone wants a quick fix—a handy pill or a fast way to avoid serious changes in the way they eat, drink, and exercise (or don't exercise). As with many of the most attractive ideas in life, this one doesn't work either. No quick fix for being out-of-shape and overweight exists.

Attempting to change your body composition by dieting alone means you must consume fewer calories than you burn each day. You expect your body to make up the deficit by converting stored body fat. In this popular notion, body fat works like a bank account. Deposit the excess, and check it out whenever you want—easy in, easy out. It seems logical: The body, having stored fat for use when needed, will burn fat exclusively and leave its muscle mass alone.

However, this view overlooks the human body's survival instinct, hard wired over the ages. In the initial stages of weight loss, muscle is at least as expendable as the precious fat reserves. The body's preference for sacrificing muscle appears stronger among the sedentary, whose bodies are trained to function with fewer and lower-quality muscle cells.

In any case, your body tenaciously resists giving up its fat reserves when you feed it less. It does this by lowering its metabolic rate so it can retain the fat for possible future survival needs. Unfortunately, the body reacts the same way whether you're ten pounds or a tenth of a ton overweight. It isn't wired to shut fat storage down, no matter how much the warehouse bulges. Loss of weight by dieting alone decreases your percentage of lean body mass and increases your percentage of body fat.

Eat better and exercise more to reduce in a healthy way. For best and quickest results, you should exercise both aerobically and to increase strength. You see, muscle burns more calories than fat 24 hours a day, so if you increase your fitness and strength, you'll burn more calories even when you aren't exercising.

However, this does not mean you have to bulk up like the Incredible Hulk with heavy weight lifting. Great progress can be made with light to moderate strength training.

Never Say Diet Again

The word *diet* has acquired a distinctly negative connotation and is often defined as a food-and-drink prescription to lose weight. But for many of us the word means *starve, thirst,* and *be miserable.* Most diets promise much and deliver little.

Going on a *diet* usually means no substantial weight loss occurs, and the dieter soon returns to old habits. Dieters even get obsessed with *tomorrow,* telling themselves, "I'll start tomorrow!" To attain and then maintain maximum velocity toward achieving your goals in your career and in your personal life, you must never think of dieting again. Diets rarely are realistic. In most cases, diets don't work, and some are even harmful to your physiology.

It comes down to this simple fact: If you don't change your eating behavior, any weight lost in dieting will, more often than not, be regained. Look at your new nutritional program as a change in status. You are upgrading your computer to process everything better so you can have a better and longer life. This is a lifestyle change to a situation where you can eat whatever you want, but just not so much of what's bad for you. Food is no longer reward or punishment—it becomes fuel to enable you to accelerate more effectively and efficiently in your profession and with your family.

Diet Dangers

Diet alone may be responsible for 35 percent of all cancer deaths, according to Food and Drug Administration reports. By the year 2000, some analysts believe research may reveal that diets are a significant causative agent in up to 60 percent of cancer deaths. Adding deaths caused by smoking to those caused by diets could then account for as much as 80 percent of all cancer deaths—if present indications are borne out by future research. This would attribute only one cancer death in five to all other factors. These should be thought-provoking numbers for overweight smokers, who are also at high risk from a different set of frequent killers: heart attacks, strokes, and other circulatory diseases.

Those numbers have a bright side. Since we are totally in control of smoking and diet, we can reduce our individual risk of developing cancer by up to 80 percent, and of dying early from circulatory diseases by a comparable percentage.

The Problem with Measuring Weight

Junk your bathroom scales. Heave them out. They're worse than useless. Let me tell you why.

Although Joe, a professional athlete, packs over 200 pounds on his under-six-foot frame, he has the "not an ounce of fat" look. Yet on some life insurance charts, he's overweight for his height. In reality he's in top shape, and his ratio of 10 percent fat to 90 percent lean body mass makes a mockery of the charts.

Robert, a professional accountant who avoids physical

exercise, is the same age, height, and weight as Joe, but Robert's corpulent body is 30 percent fat and only 70 percent lean body mass. Compared to athlete Joe, accountant Robert has to lift three times as much fat every time he stands up. He has to do it with 20 percent less lean muscle mass by volume, and with only a fraction of Joe's muscle power. No wonder Robert tires quickly.

After an ordinary day in the office, Robert goes home feeling exausted; after an ordinary day of competition or physical training, Joe is full of energy and ready to enjoy his off hours to the fullest. No wonder accountant Robert buys any diet book promising rapid weight loss without effort; no wonder he talks a good story about losing weight but never does, and no wonder walking a long way utterly exhausts him.

So throw your bathroom scales away because muscle weighs more than fat. Scales are dangerous since it's so seductively easy to think, "Numbers don't lie." Even though following the Anti-Diet program for several weeks makes you slimmer, stronger, and more energetic, unless your weight is down you can become discouraged. Some people lock onto the weight thing. In the absence of a better reading on the scale, they fail to appreciate the enormously more important fact of steadily growing leaner, healthier, and more capable.

Throwing Money at Fat

Many people throw money at their overweight condition by buying into an expensive weight-loss program. Unfortunately, this rarely gets rid of the fat permanently. In spite of all the money spent with the weight-loss industry, Americans continue to get fatter. Every generation has been getting fatter at a younger age—a frightening thought for the future.

Dieting doesn't work because it depends on deprivation. Anti-Dieting works because it increases your energy, productivity, and confidence while slimming you down and increasing your personal happiness, self-esteem, and satisfaction.

There's only one reason why anyone buys into a weight-loss program: to obtain *discipline*. If it takes paying for it to gain enough discipline to rescue your stamina and health, do it. You have too much at stake to overlook what works for you. Just make sure the program you purchase flies on both wings: (1) The program trains you to prefer, or at least to accept, foods containing fewer calories with less fat without being unrealistic over the long haul; and (2) the program provides exercise. Otherwise the extra inches around your waist or hips stick with you—only your wallet gets thinner.

The Six Principles of Anti-Dieting

Anti-Diet Principle #1: Weight doesn't matter. My experience in working with thousands of executives over many years, coupled with ongoing analysis of the scientific studies, establishes this principle beyond doubt. No controllable factor plays a more powerful role in boosting business stamina, productivity, and creativity than lowering the amount of fat, within reason, and increasing your body's lean muscle mass.

Anti-Diet Principle #2: Don't punish yourself. It's not all carrots and "rabbit food." Anti-Dieters never let themselves feel deprived; when they want a thick steak, a luscious dessert, or a candy bar, they indulge themselves. They don't feel guilty about it either because most of the time they eat smart, light, low-fat, and nutritious.

If you look on food as a pure source of simple and well-deserved pleasure, don't be put off. Most slim people enjoy food as much as heavier people do. The difference isn't in lost dining pleasure, it's in training your mind, body, and palate to enjoy nonfattening foods. Anti-Dieting is the art of enjoying nonfattening foods.

Anti-Diet Principle #3: Eat right and avoid hunger pangs. Instead of skipping meals, Anti-Dieters eat more often. They know which foods are high in calories and fat, so they consume fewer of them; they know which are low in calories and fat, so they consume more of them.

Anti-Diet Principle #4: Exercise more to prevent muscle loss. If you eat fewer calories of fat and get more exercise, you'll become leaner, more energetic, and healthier even as the years roll by. You can't slow the passage of time, but you can do a lot to shield yourself from time's attacks on your stamina. The key point here is: Just because you reduce your fat intake, you can't overindulge in calories and still control your weight.

Anti-Diet Principle #5: Train yourself to change the saturated fat food preferences you acquired as a child. Our ability to use technology to synthesize and preserve food has victimized us. Ancient humans developed a taste for fruits, berries, and the leaner game meats; today people develop a taste for chips, chocolate, and charbroiled steak. Even though many executives dine frequently in upscale restaurants, some of them have never completely shaken the food preferences they acquired before the age of twelve. I'm not saying they wish for a hamburger washed down with a cola drink when looking at the menu in a fine restaurant. Nevertheless, their subliminal bias toward high-fat food remains as strong as ever—for proof, look at their waistlines.

Anti-Diet Principle #6: Eat to recover. One of the most important concepts for new Anti-Dieters to build into their lives is recovery. Recovery is essential to the Anti-Diet program. Recovery means recapturing energy. Adequate sleep heads the list of the basic forms of recovery; adequate nutrition comes second. The list of essential recovery mechanisms goes beyond sleep and food to include water intake, humor, exercise, diversion, fun, relaxation, meditation, and even sitting down when you've been standing too long—or the reverse.

Anti-Dieters train themselves to enjoy eating in terms of recovery, rather than in terms of calorie counting, food exchanges, and the other useless mumbo-jumbo put out by the weight-loss industry. Train yourself to take care of your nutritional needs first. Developing this habit is half the battle to reaching the body size you desire.

You wouldn't put brake fluid in the gas tank of your car, or gasoline where the motor oil goes, because disaster would quickly result. In the same way, eating without regard to what your body needs causes disaster, though it will happen more slowly than doing something equally unwise to a car. So learn how to eat to replace the nutrients your body has consumed.

Learning the Language of Fitness

Anti-Dieters join a select group of thousands of corporate executives and other individuals. All of them increased their work productivity and personal happiness by learning to eat properly and exercise regularly. The Anti-Diet is a part of the Mentally Tough Corporate Training Program, presented either in-house or at the LGE corporate training facility in Orlando, Florida.

In our programs, we often use familiar words in new ways. I'll explain some of those terms now.

Corporate Athlete™ is a term I use because, to perform at high levels, a corporate executive needs as much stamina as a professional athlete needs in competitive sports. Consider the demands that today's business climate makes on Corporate Athletes: Often they must perform at highly competent levels under intense pressure for ten or more hours a day, often six days a week. They are expected to continue this extraordinary output over a career span of 30 to 40 years.

By contrast, most professional athletes are under intense practice conditions or competitive pressures for only four or five hours a day, often only during their sport's season. Moreover, sport careers typically last only three to seven years. I believe corporate executives and professional athletes have an equally great need for world-class nutrition to provide a competitive edge in the struggle for professional and personal success.

Stress, the opposite of recovery, is energy expenditure in all its forms. Two facts about stress are especially important: All forms of stress take place as biochemical events both in your mind and in your body. Emotional and mental stress is every bit as genuine as physical stress because energy is expended emotionally, mentally, and physically.

Make stress do its job. Corporate America has been sold a bill of goods about stress. It goes like this: Stress is a career-destroying monster; therefore, businesses need consultants to instruct them in stress reduction or avoidance methods.

Not true!

Here's what we've learned about stress: Avoiding stress reduces functional capacity, and seeking stress helps you reach your highest potential.

In my view, we have all heard far too much about stress reduction, about people being "stressed out," and about the severe stresses of numerous activities. There are only two reasons you ever feel "stressed out": (1) Your capacity for stress is not high enough, or (2) you are not getting enough recovery.

You can train to increase your capacity to deal with heightened stress; you can also train to perform at even higher levels under the heightened stress. The truth is, *in and of itself,* stress not only is harmless, it's essential to growth, to greater achievement, and to life itself. The central concept of stress is this: *Stress only becomes dangerous when it's not balanced by appropriate and adequate recovery.*

Many things can cause stress in some situations and recovery in others. For example, sitting too long is a form of stress; on the other hand, sitting down after being on your feet too long is recovery.

Ideal Performance State™ (IPS) is the most effective and reliable mental, emotional, and physical state for performing at your highest level. Corporate Athletes experience a specific group of positive feelings and emotions when they are in IPS: challenged, energized, and confident with a sense of joy, fun, and fulfillment. Someone in business may speak of "being on a roll" when talking about how they felt when in IPS. In sports, the popular term is "in the zone."

Recovery is anything that recaptures energy—such as sleep, adequate nutrition, exercise, humor, active and passive rest, need fulfilment, and social interaction. It is essential to balance stress with recovery.

Ideal Recovery State™ (IRS) is a situation you achieve for recapturing energy so you can continue to perform at high levels. IRS involves feelings of openness, peacefulness, calm, reduced anxiety, re-energizing, etc.

Mental Toughness refers to a dynamic state of being in which the tough person meets stress with a flexible and responsive attitude characterized by strength and resiliency. Being Mentally Tough® means you can access IPS (if you are in a performance mode) even under the most difficult circumstances.

Why Does the Body Store Fat?

Some paleoanthropologists believe our genes and bodies have developed into their present form over the past 70 million years. But refrigerators have been with us for less than a century—in other words, our pervasive technological civilization has not had time to make a dent in our bodies' hard-wired survival reactions. On a larger scale, the agricultural revolution freed much of humanity from depending on hunting and gathering for their daily food. It began no more than a mere 10,000 years ago.

Comparing 70 million to 10 thousand gives us some idea why our bodies cling so stubbornly to their ancient distrust that food will always be easily obtained. They cling also to their ancient conviction that survival depends on storing fat against future famine. This echo of our primitive past has long outlived its usefulness in the industrialized West, but modern science has found no way to silence it.

We can, however, influence our bodies' constant urge to store fat. Here are some do's and don'ts:

- *Do* eat five or six small meals a day so you never feel really hungry.
- *Do* eat a variety of foods to reduce your chances of having a deficiency in some area.
- *Do* exercise more, both aerobically and for strength, but never when you're weak with hunger. If you're hungry before a workout, eat an apple or some other convenient fresh fruit, vegetable, or grain product.
- *Do* build more physical activity into your daily routine. It isn't easy in our hurry-up, mechanized society, but be alert to exercises you can integrate into your daily activities. Many times they can be time-savers.
- *Do* organize your life to seek—rather than avoid—physical exertion. You can fit it in if you give it high priority. Exercise is too important to let slide because you think you can't find the time to preserve your health. If you don't, who will?
- *Do* minimize your intake of simple sugars.
- *Don't* skip a meal to compensate for overeating. Doing so trains your body to store fat more aggressively.

 • *Don't* eat only one or two meals a day. Either one is another feast and famine routine that trains your body to store fat.

Knowing how to improve your ratio of lean body mass-to-fat is the first step toward achieving permanent weight loss. The second step is to develop sufficient motivation to carry you through to your goal. Effective techniques for increasing your motivation to energize your life through Anti-Dieting appear in the following chapters.

Let's not overlook one more vital benefit of adopting the Anti-Diet lifestyle: By drastically reducing all the controllable risk factors known today, Anti-Dieting adds years to your life, and life to your years.

Chapter 2

WHERE ARE YOU STARTING FROM?

"Getting rich and sick is stupid."
—Tom Hopkins (referring to how people devote so much time to their career that their health is sacrificed)

On a recent early morning flight from Philadelphia to my office in Orlando, the flight attendant handed out what was called a "breakfast snack." It was a container holding a small box of Total cereal, some low-fat milk, and a slice of banana nut bread.

"Hey," I thought, "this isn't bad."

The gentleman across the aisle had a different reaction. He said the snack wasn't what he wanted. He asked for a Danish— one of those jelly-filled doughnuts with about 24 grams of saturated fat. Our gracious flight attendant said she didn't have any. Hearing this, the gentleman asked her to check the first-class section because, "A Danish is what I want."

She dutifully came back after checking first class and recited their menu: oatmeal, low-fat milk, and fruit. The gentleman burst out in a frustrated tone, "Who ever heard of an airline not serving a Danish! That's how I start my day."

Yes, he was overweight, and probably slowly but steadily gaining weight. After all, he had the ghosts of countless Danishes past jiggling under his skin. But I didn't say anything. Obviously he wasn't ready for my message. All I could do was hope for lifestyle wisdom to catch up with him before a heart attack.

Americans Diet More, But Are More Obese

The French spend far more time thinking and talking about food than Americans do. The Dutch spend a far higher percentage of income on food than we do. Yet only in Samoa can a higher percentage of obesity be found among the general population. We can't argue that a harsh climate keeps Americans indoors and prevents them from exercising (although climate certainly is a factor in New England, the Midwest, and the states bordering Canada). This excuse falls apart when we consider the Scandinavians who, even though they have brutal winters, have far more cross-country skiers and, in summer, far more bicycle riders. And for at least two decades, the Japanese have been rich enough to eat as poorly as we do; and yet, except for sumo wrestlers, few Japanese are seriously overweight.

As a nation, we eat too much fat and often way too many carbohydrates. We consume too many poor-quality calories, and we don't exercise enough. Most of us have very few unavoidable physical demands built into our lives, and more labor-saving gadgets come on the market every year. Human muscle now provides only a tiny fraction of the effort required to produce and distribute goods as more Americans earn their livings in sedentary pursuits.

This is a worldwide phenomenon; the United States merely leads the parade. In time, the rest of the world will catch up to us in eliminating built-in exercise from daily life. We know they are already doing so because obesity rates are on the rise throughout the industrialized world.

We are now in our second generation of couch potatoes, and TV is no longer the lone culprit. Computers and home video games are spreading even more rear ends across chairs and floors in America.

Is Being Overweight a Mark of Success?

In parts of the third world, being corpulent is still a mark of success. In those countries, only rich people can afford the indolence and food it takes to get fat. In such places one often sees the fat bigshot with a flock of skinny groupies surrounding his or her ponderous dignity.

Even in the industrialized West, men with a balcony of fat overhanging their belts sometimes joke about how much their fat verandas cost them. "Thousands of hard-earned dollars went right here," they'll say, patting their bulging bellies. Or, "It took more than 50 head of prime Texas beef to build this monument to my success." It virtually becomes their cathedral of corpulence.

In this country the prevalence of obesity, even among people on welfare, has robbed excessive stoutness of its éclat. Rather than indicating individual wealth, obesity among the low-income segment of the American population is a manifestation of national wealth in material terms—and of national poverty in intellectual, rational, and educational terms.

Being overweight never gained wide acceptance as a status symbol in this country. On the contrary, everyone, including the obese, has long known what a deadly curse being fat is. Still, along with our high rates of obesity, we have attendant high rates of degenerative disease and premature death among people in the prime of life. We also have a high incidence of, and a high death rate from, anorexia nervosa—an eating disorder triggered primarily by starvation and malnutrition.

The Cost of the Weight Epidemic

Near the end of 1994, the *New York Times* published an article headlined, "The U.S. Is Now Fatter Than Ever." It reported that not only is American obesity at an all-time high, but it is taking place when awareness has never been greater and despite the exponential growth of the diet industry (now estimated at $50 billion annually). The article also reported that obesity among children is increasing at an even faster rate than among adults.

In an editorial in the *Journal of the American Medical Association*, F. Xavier Pisunyen, Professor of Medicine at Columbia University, wrote, "The proportion of the population that is obese is incredible. If this was about tuberculosis, it would be called an epidemic."

In a scientific journal called *Pharmaco Economics*, Graham Colditz of the Harvard University School of Medicine set the 1990 obesity cost to our nation at $68.8 billion.

What Is Overweight and Overfat?

The famous life insurance charts (developed about 1935) list acceptable weights for men and women of various ages and heights. Their unique characteristic is their breakdown of acceptable weights for each height into small, medium, and large body frame calories. Although the instructions with the charts detail how to measure your frame size, most overweight people go right to the "Large Frame" column because the weights are higher.

Overfat implies you are simply carrying more fat than you should. If you would so describe yourself, it's time to make changes in your lifestyle through good nutrition (not dieting) and exercise.

For women, having 27 percent or more of body fat is a good marker for being overfat; for men the number is 20 percent.

Obesity is defined as storing excess fat as a reserve. Few sources give an exact body fat percentage at which we can say someone is obese, but a woman with over 32 percent and a man with over 25 percent body fat would be approaching obesity.

Regardless of your current ratio of body fat to lean body mass, you should give high priority to reaching the ideal ratios. Ideally, a woman's body fat will be under 22 percent and a man's under 17 percent. However, you must have some fat, both on your body and in your diet. Women should never allow their body fat to go below 12 percent; men should avoid dropping below 5 percent. Although there are cases of athletes of both genders being under those minimums, they should be the exception, not the rule.

Watching the Right Gauges

Imagine that a steam locomotive engineer knows he has a faulty safety valve, which affects the engine's team pressure. Do you think he'd spend most of his time checking on the coal supply instead of watching the steam pressure gauge? No, he'd keep his eye glued to the steam pressure gauge, wouldn't he? His main concern would be to make sure the rising pressure in the boiler wouldn't blow up.

Similarly, we all have the equivalent of a steam pressure

gauge to protect us from excess body fat. It's not the bathroom scale, which often gives misleading readings. There's an equally convenient method you only need do once a month. All it takes is a cloth tape measure and a few minutes.

Measure your thigh at its midsection, and at your waist just below the navel. Apply just enough tension to the tape to hold it horizontally. Do this once a month and record the results so you will be encouraged by your progress. These measurements give you a better insight into your health and fitness than weighing yourself every day.

What Is Your Body Fat Percentage?

Your body fat can be measured in many ways. Many universities and hospitals throughout the world have underwater weighing machines. You put on a swimsuit and are submerged while breathing through an apparatus. After you exhale as much as you can, your body is weighed and the device measures your density relative to the density of water. It can tell you within one percent what your body fat percentage is.

Some doctors, hospital staffs, and university researchers use skinfold calipers to measure the thickness of the fat underneath the skin. Mathematical equations convert the caliper reading to body fat percentage, yielding a result within two percent of the reading obtained by the water immersion method.

You can also use inexpensive plastic skinfold calipers to measure yourself. Researchers find that plastic skinfold calipers are adequate for personal assessment. Although they are still in development, these devices are probably better than relying on your bathroom scale.*

Many people climb on the scales in the morning only to moan, "No dessert for me today." Some get on the scales and say, "Yes! I can have dessert." Some people's lives revolve around their bathroom scale. But the scale focuses their attention on the wrong things.

Can you eat anything you want? You'll soon say you can if you commit to the Anti-Diet program. If you eat intelligently,

---

*Please contact LGE Sport Science at 1-800-543-7764 to obtain a skinfold caliper.

you can eat almost anything you want when you want it. All it takes to reach this pleasant state is to make good nutrition decisions most of the time. The Anti-Diet program can get you there, though you have to make some performance and health-building decisions and stick to them. What works is to change your lifestyle.

It's not necessary to become fanatic about it. Just begin moving steadily away from bad food choices and no exercise toward good food choices and increased exercise. Let your mind and body adjust to your new direction before putting the pedal to the metal.

For the first month or two—longer if you're overfat, over 40, or under-exercised—be content to make a little progress every day. Especially, avoid the "no pain, no gain" philosophy because it sidelines thousands of eager exercisers with injuries. Commit to making one positive change a week; get comfortable with this schedule before you increase the pace of change.

Begin by recording your present body measurements so you can be encouraged by your progress as time passes. Just one more caution: Don't celebrate an improvement in health and leanness with a food binge. Reward yourself, sure, but do it with moderation, as befits the new priority you've set for yourself: to reach the highest possible velocity toward achieving your maximum potential in your career and in your personal life.

How Long Does It Take to Get There?

No simple, hard-and-fast rule can cover how much time it takes to reach the ideal ratio of body fat to lean body mass. Consider these two individuals: First, a 24-year-old moderately active woman in good health with 27 percent body fat; second, a 56-year-old sedentary man in poor health whose body fat is 35 percent. How rapidly each person changes depends totally on age, gender, activity level, and body fat percentage. Therefore, each person has different needs to consider before setting goals for improved health and nutrition.

Those who set out to increase the level of exercise in their lives should obtain a doctor's approval first, but this is especially important for anyone who has any heart or circulatory ailment, a serious chronic condition, is over 30 years old, or is more than 5 percentage points over ideal body fat.

Regardless of how much body fat you need to lose and how much muscle you need to increase, please remember: It's going to take time! Unfortunately, people get warped in their thinking about how fast they can make these changes in their body's composition.

Recently I was traveling by airplane, sitting next to a somewhat eccentric but pleasant lady in her mid-30s. Without knowing what I did for a living, she began extolling the virtues of her personal trainer, and how he had done wonders with her. She went on and on, explaining his breadth of knowledge and his manner of training. Following his guidance, she had lost two percent of her body fat. He sounded too good to be true. And he was!

When I asked how long they had been working together, she said, "One week!" My jaw dropped, and I asked, "How did he measure you? What were his goals for you? Was he the one who said you had lost two percent fat?"

He used skinfold calipers, which have a slight measurement error anyway. But he was misinformed about body fat, so he misinformed her. Gently, I explained how a two percent decrease in body fat in one week is nearly impossible. I discovered he was not a certified personal trainer, and she thanked me for going into such detail to discuss the issue. I'm not sure if she fired her trainer or just rationalized that his calipers were broken, but at least I felt better knowing she understood more about her body.

Analyzing Your Present Food Intake

How do you go about reorganizing your diet to meet those objectives so that you can get on with achieving your maximum potential? The first step is to analyze what you're eating now. Log what and when you eat and drink for two days. Carry a little notebook and jot down what, when, and how much as you consume food and drink. Include everything: a cup of coffee and the sugar and cream that you put in it. Also include any cans of soda you down, and your water intake from all sources. The more accurately you report this, the more accurate the analysis will be. Take your two-day log to any certified nutritionist for analysis.

If you like, I will respond with an analysis of what you're

now eating and give you my recommendations for what your total caloric intake should be, along with how you can improve your diet to increase your stamina and energy.*

How Healthy Is Your Diet?

You might need about 2,000 calories a day, depending on your gender, height, weight, age, how active you are, and what your body composition is right now. For the moment, let's go with 2,000 calories a day. My recommendation is that the 2,000 calories should be divided as follows: Aim to eat about one-third more and up to equal amounts of carbohydrates—fruits, grains, and vegetables—as you do of protein in seafood, poultry, and red meat. Eat a small amount of red meat no more than twice a week. If you do that, you shouldn't have any trouble meeting your fat requirement.

How healthy is your diet? When I ask corporate executives to give me their perceptions of their diet, on the average, about 50 percent give their diets a 7 or above on the 10-point scale—10 being very healthy, 1 being unhealthy. Others give their diets a 6 or less, so I estimate that over half of the Corporate Athletes I address rate their nutrition as so-so at best.

Knowing How Much to Eat

If he's doing absolutely nothing, a man uses about 11 calories per pound of body weight every 24 hours just to keep breathing. A woman needs about 10 calories per pound because her body typically has less muscle. A mostly sedentary office job burns 40 or 50 percent more. Running 20 miles a week would only take an additional 500 or 600 calories per week, or about 70 to 85 more calories a day. So it's easy to overestimate how much you can eat to compensate for high activity.

Your daily allotment of fat is between 33 and 50 grams of fat. This is what's allowed if you have a 2,000 calorie diet. Let's work with about the upper middle portion of the range: 44 grams of fat. You can get that fat anywhere you want, but preferably from fish and plants.

---

*See the appendix for information on how to obtain your nutritional analysis.

Although the key element to control in your food intake is fat, it's important not to go overboard and try to eliminate fat from your diet. To function, your body must have some fat. Eating excessive amounts of fat, particularly saturated fat, is what does the damage.

How Many Calories Do You Need?

Once you know what you need to stay where you are, your level of control improves. If you are now slightly plump, and drop your average daily caloric intake by 100 calories of fat (that's slightly over 11 grams) and expand slightly on your present activity level, you will probably change your body composition (your ratio of body fat to lean body mass) a little each month. This comfortable rate allows your skin to adjust and avoids or minimizes wrinkle formation.

If you are now more than slightly plump, or want quicker results, drop your average caloric intake by more than 100 calories (the best calories to drop are the high-fat ones) and expand your physical activity considerably.

If you're accelerating your physical activity, you should expand the protein component of your diet to support an increase in muscle mass.

You can zero in on the fat component of your diet, and substitute lower fat or nonfat items (just watch out for the sugar in some fat-free foods) so you can lose weight without feeling hungry.

Seven Maintenance Diets

Here are seven examples of maintenance diets for men and women of different ages, weights, and activity levels. Probably you can find one similar to your situation. Remember: a *sedentary* person is an inactive couch potato, possibly allergic to exercise. A *moderately active* person is on his or her feet much of the day and exercises only about two hours each week. A *very active* person gets at least six hours of vigorous aerobic exercise and strength work per week.

- A sedentary 40-year-old woman, who is 5 feet 7 inches tall and weighs 130 pounds, needs only 1,695 calories a day to maintain body weight. Eating more calories causes weight gain unless they're burned off by increased exercise.

• A moderately active 30-year-old woman, who is 5 feet 2 inches tall and weighs 105 pounds, needs only 1,983 calories a day to maintain body weight, but she can consume more calories without gaining weight if she becomes very active. As a very active person, her daily requirements to maintain body weight would shoot up to 2,727 calories a day.

• A very active 50-year-old woman, who is 5 feet 11 inches tall and weighs 140 pounds, needs 2,482 calories a day to maintain body weight.

• A very active 30-year-old woman, who is 5 feet 2 inches tall and 105 pounds, must eat 2,800 calories a day to maintain her body weight.

• A sedentary 25-year-old man, 5 feet 6 inches tall and weighing 200 pounds, on average can eat no more than 2,599 calories a day. Otherwise, he will gain weight unless he exercises enough to burn his excess calories. If he diets without exercise, he may lose some pounds, but the fat component of his fat-muscle ratio will increase.

• A moderately active 45-year-old man, who is 5 feet 10 inches tall and weighs 175 pounds, needs only 1,983 calories a day to maintain his body weight.

• A very active 58-year-old man, 6 feet tall and weighing 160 pounds, needs 3,134 calories a day to maintain his body weight.

These seven daily cases are plotted on the following chart according to weight. Four variables important in determining

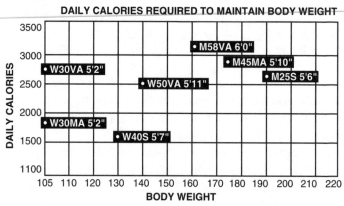

DAILY CALORIES REQUIRED TO MAINTAIN BODY WEIGHT

daily maintenance requirements are given for each example—gender, age, activity level (S, sedentary; MA, moderately active; VA, very active), and height.

The first person listed (shown as W40 S 5' 7" on the chart) is a woman, 40 years old, sedentary, and 5 feet 7 inches tall.

The Nutrition Analysis

While attending an executive seminar, a woman reported this diet: *Breakfast:* one slice of white bread toast with butter and cheese and one cup of coffee. *Lunch:* a small portion of lean beef, 2 cups mixed vegetables, 3 small potatoes, and a sparkling water. *Dinner:* 2 slices of bread and 2 pieces of sausage pizza.

Analysis of this active executive's diet revealed that she consumed 1,400 calories: 57 grams of protein, 227 grams of carbohydrates, and 32 grams of total fat. The calories are way too low. Total fat is also low, but the saturated fat component (from the butter, cheese, beef, and pizza) is much too high. If she's active she will improve her body composition, but I would worry greatly about her health. To avoid health problems she should increase her consumption of quality calories. Eating a diet high in saturated fat and low in calories can cause degenerative diseases to develop over time.

In a different seminar, another woman recorded this diet: *Breakfast:* half a banana, healthy grain cereal, low-fat milk, fresh juice, and one cup of coffee. *Lunch:* a glass of milk, an apple, cashews, decaffeinated coffee, and light tuna on whole wheat bread with light mayonnaise. *Dinner:* pasta with tomato sauce, apple juice, a cookie, and coffee with low-fat milk.

She had consumed 2,200 calories, which is 111 percent of where she should be. She had a lot of protein, and the carbohydrates were excellent, but the fat was a little too high. This person need not change her diet much because she has a healthy mix of vitamins and minerals.

For breakfast, one of the men ate a whole-wheat roll with preserves, orange juice, and coffee with sugar and milk. At lunch, he had a roast beef and cheese sandwich on whole wheat bread, mineral water, brewed coffee, and a cookie. For dinner, he ate steak and a baked potato with cheese along with three beers.

This gentleman put away 2,000 calories, which is only 66 percent of what he should have eaten for the day. He had 83 grams of protein and 63 grams of fat, which is too high. He needs to substitute more complex carbohydrates such as rice, other vegetables, and whole grains for some of the fatty foods and eliminate at least two of the beers.

Another man had grain cereal, melon, coffee, and whole wheat toast with butter and jam in the morning. *Lunch:* soup, baked fish, salad with light dressing, mineral water, citrus fruit juice, coffee, and a slice of angel food cake. *Dinner:* baked chicken with spaghetti, tossed green salad with dressing, and bread.

This man did pretty well. He ate almost 3,000 calories, but he's extremely active. He only had 89 percent of what he was supposed to consume. His total fat was a little too high. His diet for the day was pretty healthy from the nutritional standpoint of vitamins and minerals. If he makes some changes on his carbohydrate and fat intake, this gentleman will be right on target.

Jane Stanfield, a 40-year-old woman who weighs 128 pounds, is 5 feet 5 inches tall. Jane is moderately active, so she should eat 2,074 calories a day: 130 grams of protein, 285 grams of carbohydrates, and 46 grams of fat.

Her husband, John, also 40 years old, is 6 feet tall and weighs 185 pounds. Since he is also moderately active, he should consume about 3,027 calories a day, drawn from 189 grams of protein, 417 grams of carbohydrate, and 67 grams of fat.

These recommendations will keep them both right where they are in body weight as long as they remain moderately active.

By changing your diet just a little bit, you can make major changes in your life. Here's what I recommend for you: Eat more lean proteins such as egg whites, skinless chicken, skinless turkey, lean red meat such as veal, and fish; more fruits and vegetables; more salads with little or no dressing; more potatoes and whole-grain breads; more low-sugar cereals such as oatmeal and Cream of Wheat; and more yogurt. Eat fresh food as often as possible, and drink lots of fruit juices. Have your meats and fish broiled or grilled rather than fried.

The Where-Are-You-Starting-from Questionnaire

Answer **True** or **False** for each question.

1. Broiled, steamed, and baked are low-fat terms.
2. The most important nutrient you can consume is water.
3. Fat is a major source of energy.
4. There is no ideal body weight or fat-to-muscle ratio for a particular individual.
5. You should eat a small meal at least two hours before facing a major performance test (a crucial meeting or negotiation, making an important presentation, giving a speech).
6. The words *lite* and *lean* on a label mean the food is healthier.
7. Most red meat is high in fat.
8. You should get most of your energy from carbohydrates.
9. The skin on a chicken breast is mostly fat and contains more than 100 calories.
10. Raw vegetables are better for you than cooked vegetables.
11. Sugar can make you hyperactive or out of control.
12. You can become addicted to sugar.
13. Honey has the same effect on you as sugar.
14. You should wait until you're thirsty to take a drink of water.
15. A vitamin and mineral supplement is probably appropriate for active people of any age, regardless of their diet.
16. Active people need to consume fat.
17. The fried fish at most fast-food restaurants is higher in calories than hamburger.
18. The sugar found in fruit is nutritionally good for you, and you can have as much as you want.
19. Cholesterol is found only in meats, dairy products, and other animal food products.
20. Protein and fat cause food to stay in the stomach longer.
21. Vitamins and minerals are major sources of energy.

Answers

1. True	7. True	13. True	19. True
2. True	8. True	14. False	20. True
3. False	9. True	15. True	21. False
4. True	10. True	16. True	
5. True	11. False	17. True	
6. False	12. False	18. False	

Evaluating Your Score

18 or more correct—You possess excellent nutritional knowledge, but are you committed to using this knowledge in your daily life?

15 to 17 correct—You're doing okay, but make sure you keep your commitment up.

14 or fewer correct—You need to improve your nutritional knowledge. Improving your diet is difficult if you're not more aware of your nutritional needs.

Chapter 3

STRATEGIC EATING AND SNACKING

"A bite in time saves nine."
(with apologies to) Benjamin Franklin

The Anti-Diet is about changing the eating habits of America. They need a lot of work. Many Americans skip breakfast and eat a hurried lunch, often with some high-fat snacks in between. Then they go home to a late evening dinner. Sound familiar? If you're eating like this, you're not fueling your mind or body to achieve maximum potential.

The Anti-Diet plan for nutrition is simple and straightforward: Eat for sustainable high performance, health, and longevity. Doing that means minimizing your consumption of red meat, fried foods, saturated fat, highly processed foods, sugary foods and drinks, and alcohol. It means maximizing your consumption of fruits, vegetables, whole-grain cereals and breads, fish, poultry, and nature's gift to power performance: pure water.

It also means eating more often: four to six small meals a day instead of three or fewer. It means timing your meals so you avoid sugar spikes and troughs, so you never feel weak with hunger, so you never tell your body to slow your metabolism because famine is on the way, and so you're brimming with energy throughout your active day.

And it means never eating a huge meal. Consuming too much food at one time interrupts your eating and elimination rhythm and tends to cause you to skip a following meal. Worse yet, if you load your huge meal with fat, which often happens with huge meals, the amount of fat in your bloodstream can shoot up to dangerously high levels.

41

Specific Recommendations

Let's now focus on what to eat and what to minimize. I'll start with the positive half of the equation:

Eat or Drink:
- Fruits
- Vegetables, particularly the green leafy varieties
- Salads, pasta, rice, whole-grain breads, oatmeal and other cereals that have no added sugar
- Salad dressings based on olive oil, or nonfat dressings
- Egg whites, plain yogurt
- Grilled, baked or barbecued turkey and chicken (without skin)
- Fish and seafood
- Water
- Pure fruit juices (no sugar added)
- Baked, broiled, or grilled meats
- Lean cuts of meat

Eat or Drink Moderately:
- Fatty red meat, no matter how it is cooked
- Fried poultry
- Fried seafood
- Fried vegetables
- Butter, mayonnaise
- Creamy salad dressings: Ranch, French, Bleu Cheese, Thousand Island, Creamy Italian
- Egg yolks, ice cream, doughnuts, Danishes, cookies, candy
- Soft drinks and alcoholic beverages
- Coffee

Minimize:
- Margarine
- Simple sugars

Fanatic Deprivation Is Counterproductive

I've heard and seen hundreds of cases of people falling off the health-food wagon. Many hands go up when I ask the audience if they know someone who binged on food after following a strict diet for some time. (Fewer hands go up if I ask whether *they* ever binge.)

The worst case was a world-class athlete I worked with in 1987. Extremely aware of nutrition, this great performer would only buy foods in the health sections of supermarkets, and she was meticulous about how they were cooked.

One day she came into my office on the verge of tears and told me about her just-eaten lunch. After a great workout in the morning, she felt good about herself and decided that a nice lunch at a restaurant was in order. She told me that she went to the salad bar and had potato salad, bean salad, and coleslaw. She then waited for my response. It wasn't as negative as she expected.

Of course, she knew about the high-fat content of those foods (the mayonnaise). I told her she could have eaten better, but it was all right to consume foods now and then that please the palate but otherwise aren't so good.

Stopping me in midsentence, she said, "I went back for seconds on everything."

Because of her awareness and honesty, there was no way I could speak negatively to her. She went on, "I've got to get it all out in the open," and told me she'd had two pieces of chocolate pie. Then, on the way back to practice, she had stopped at a convenience market for two double-stuffed cookies, a Snickers, and a pint of skim milk, all of which she had wolfed down.

This is an extreme example of someone who needed help to correct a problem, but her case serves as an excellent introduction to this concept.

To raise your energy to the next level, you must be honest with yourself and face the truth. Setting eating goals more strict than you can sustain puts you at great risk of falling into the yo-yo diet trap. This is the direct opposite of the Anti-Diet program, which calls for intelligent commitment and the sensible retraining of habits rather than unsustainable deprivation.

The Three-Meals-a-Day Mind-Set

Most of us get locked into the three-meals-a-day mind-set. It's no wonder. After all, it's traditional to eat breakfast, lunch and dinner. Somewhere, we were told if we ate less (in amount, duration, and frequency) we would lose weight. Today, nutritional science gives us incredible insight into these concepts.

We now know the physiological effects of eating (or not eating) three meals a day. Skipping breakfast and eating nothing before noon means your brain is starved of its principal fuel (glucose) until lunchtime. Clearly, you'll be at your productive peak only for a time after lunch—and then only if you don't eat a large, fat-heavy, drowsiness-producing meal.

The day gets off to a far better start if you eat breakfast early in the morning. However, on the three-meal plan, you will have a rise in blood sugar, but by late morning your blood sugar will

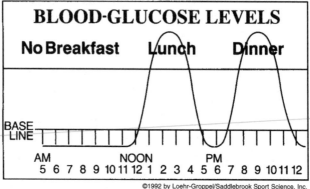

BLOOD-GLUCOSE LEVELS

No Breakfast   Lunch   Dinner

BASE LINE

AM   NOON   PM
5 6 7 8 9 10 11 12 1 2 3 4 5 6 7 8 9 10 11 12

©1992 by Loehr-Groppel/Saddlebrook Sport Science, Inc.

drop back so much that you will be definitely in a depressed blood-sugar state. The same occurs in the late afternoon.

Both slumps can be headed off since the brain works on glucose. One simple way to head off blood-sugar troughs is to eat a small snack in the midmorning and another in the

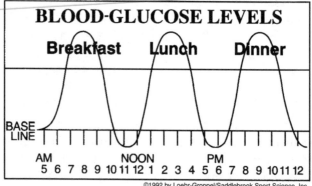

BLOOD-GLUCOSE LEVELS

Breakfast   Lunch   Dinner

BASE LINE

AM   NOON   PM
5 6 7 8 9 10 11 12 1 2 3 4 5 6 7 8 9 10 11 12

©1992 by Loehr-Groppel/Saddlebrook Sport Science, Inc.

midafternoon. This serves to stabilize your blood-sugar levels, enabling you to be more cognitive throughout the day.

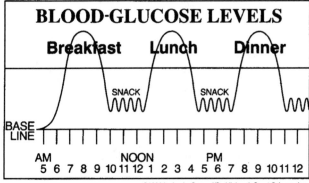

©1992 by Loehr-Groppel/Saddlebrook Sport Science, Inc.

Setting Yourself Up for a Productive Day

The setup is called breakfast. Break the fast imposed by sleep and refuel your mind and body. It's not a new concept. The term *breakfast* dates from the 15th century, and the concept probably became well established during or even before the earliest civilizations. It's hard to imagine a gang of pyramid builders setting out on empty stomachs to pull huge blocks of granite across the Egyptian desert. But every generation has to learn the importance of breakfast for itself.

You may get up in a fog and hate the idea of eating, but, as always, your body remains in a survival mode. It won't release the muscles' limited store of energy in case some sudden emergency requires fight or flight. All our progress in civilization has not ruled out that possibility.

If you eat a high-carbohydrate diet, you replace the glycogen (or starch) in the liver much more quickly than if you eat a protein and fat diet. Protein and fat replace glycogen slowly; carbohydrates replace glycogen quickly. Specifically, whole-grain breads and cereals, such as oatmeal, provide a far more productive breakfast for a mental worker than ham and eggs.

The body wants to be energized when it awakens. Research shows that most people reach their highest level of mental energy within six hours of waking up. A protein breakfast won't necessarily make you more alert; a carbohydrate breakfast won't necessarily make you calmer. However, eating something for breakfast is essential to give your blood glucose levels a jump start.

We know food helps wake us up. After sleeping, your body's glycogen supplies are at their lowest level, and the physical processes need a kick start. The brain works on two things: oxygen and glucose. With little oxygen, you die. With little glucose, you sleep. With little glycogen available for conversion into glucose and no breakfast, you tend to function cognitively way below your best.

People who perform below their potential all morning are likely to say: "I don't have time to eat breakfast." Missing breakfast is often a characteristic of someone who flails away frantically, working hard without accomplishing much.

Even the busiest person can find a few moments between getting up and getting to work to make a breakfast of bananas, oatmeal, rye toast, bran muffins, or bagels, even if there isn't time for a quick bowl of cereal topped with fruit.

Healthy Breakfasts for Maximum Stamina

Here's what people typically eat for breakfast. To gain maximum mental, emotional, and physical stamina, you must combine the right amounts of protein and carbohydrates.

Recommend Often:

Food	Cal.	Carb.	Prot.	Sat. Fat	Unsat. Fat	Fiber	Sugar
Apple (medium)	81	21	.26	.08	.17	2.9	18.1 (fructose*)
Cereal, TOTAL™ (1cup)	116	26	3.3	.1	.41	3.5	3.5
2% Milk	121	11.7	8.1	2.9	1.21	0	11.7
Toast (rye, unbuttered, 2 slices)	141	25.6	4.96	.5	1.4	2.6	2.2
Orange Juice (8 oz.)	102	23.6	1.6	.05	.17	.45	23.1 (fructose*)
Potatoes (1 serving of breakfast potatoes)	49.2	11.4	1.1	.02	.03	.85	.57
Egg substitutes	47.4	.36	6.8	.38	1.4	0	.36
Pancakes (no butter)	104	19.8	2.8	.27	.74	.75	4.5

* Fructose is the natural sugar found in fruits that enters the bloodstream so slowly that sugar spikes never result.

Not Recommended (high in saturated fat and cholesterol):

Food	Cal.	Carb.	Prot.	Sat. Fat	Unsat. Fat	Fiber	Sugar
Buttered Toast (white bread, 2 tablespoons butter, two slices)	209	25.6	5.0	5.3	8.4	2.6	2.2
2 Eggs (scrambled)	202	2.7	13.5	4.5	8.4	0	2.7
Ham	239	2.8	19	4.9	9.2	0	2.9
2 Pancakes (short stack with butter and syrup)	391	65.7	7.1	4.4	5.2	.23	45.3
3 Pancakes (full stack with butter and syrup)	587	98.6	10.7	6.7	9.3	.24	68
1 Waffle (with butter and syrup)	489	69.3	6.1	9.3	11.4	1.1	30.8

Find Time to Eat Breakfast

People are always telling me they don't have time to eat breakfast. I can't say this strongly enough: *Eat Breakfast.* Period. No ifs, ands, or buts.

A good night's sleep depletes much of the glycogen stored in the liver. (Glycogen is the starch the body converts to glucose for energy.)

The brain works on two things, oxygen and glucose. With the storage bin containing the glycogen fairly well depleted in the morning, you must eat something for breakfast to function at a high level. It can be a small breakfast; it can be a quick breakfast, but food intake can't be omitted entirely without gravely weakening your morning's productivity.

As an aside for those who study physiology and know that glycogen is also stored in the muscles, I offer this theory: The body won't utilize muscle glycogen unless we are literally starving.

Still no time to eat breakfast? As several studies show, eating breakfast is associated with improved midmorning endurance and with better attitudes toward work.

Still no time? How about some ready-to-eat foods? Apples, yogurt, whole-grain muffins, and bagels are just a few examples of foods you can eat on the run, driving a car, whatever.

If you don't eat breakfast, I urge you in the strongest terms to reconsider your position. From the viewpoint of losing fat, it's imperative. If you don't eat breakfast every morning you tell your body in loud and clear tones: "I'm starving. Do something to save my life." Your body responds by lowering its metabolism and energy output to store more fat.

There is simply no reason to avoid eating in the morning. Breakfast is not the time to "Just say no!"

Insulin: The Real Reason You Could Be Storing More Fat

For many of us, we associate insulin with diabetes. But contemporary nutritional science demands that we pay close attention to the issues behind what and when we eat, the type of food we consume, the speed of that food's ability to increase blood sugar, the subsequent response of insulin, and finally, the role of insulin in either burning that blood sugar or storing it as fat. I know that sounds like a lot of "stuff" to concern yourself with, but believe me, it's possible this may be your most important lesson in nutrition. It could mean the difference between health and sickness, lean versus overfat, and content versus discontent.

Insulin is a hormone associated with energy abundance. It is secreted by the pancreas. Its primary responsibility is to stabilize the sugar level in your blood, but it does much more than that. We know today that when you consume a lot of high-energy foods (e.g., carbohydrates), insulin is secreted in great abundance. When you consume excess carbohydrates, they are first stored as glycogen in the muscles and liver. But as soon as the liver and muscle glycogen stores are full (which doesn't take much), insulin stimulates the conversion of blood sugar to fat.

Insulin plays a very specific role in the body's metabolism, and this purpose is so important that I feel today's Corporate Athletes should know what happens when they eat certain foods. The primary job of insulin is to increase the use of glucose by the body. That, initially, decreases how the body uses fat. At the same time, insulin also promotes the development of fatty acids. This is what happens: Insulin first sends glucose to the liver. Once the liver's glycogen level reaches a 5 to 6 percent concentration (not too much, is it?), the storage of glycogen stops there. If you exercise after eating a meal, some glucose is transported to the muscle, but your muscles can only store about a 2 percent concentration of glycogen (again, not too much). If the storage depots are full, all extra glucose will be converted to fat. If you are active and your storage depots are depleted, glucose can feed the muscles to keep them working.

Insulin also facilitates the transport of amino acids to the cells after proteins are broken down. When associated with growth hormones, insulin increases the capability of amino acids to penetrate the cells. Insulin also inhibits the breakdown of proteins within the cells, especially muscle cells. Therefore, amino acids are released from these cells less frequently. So insulin promotes the formation of protein within cells, but prevents protein breakdown inside the cells.

Keeping an Even Keel

The current thinking is that the ratio of carbohydrates to protein should never go above two to one. Once it does, insulin production increases rapidly. The ideal is to consume one third more or nearly equal amounts of carbohydrates than you consume of protein, and to minimize your intake of simple sugars. Also, make sure that the protein you consume comes from low-fat sources. Your fat intake should be about one fifth of your diet, and the fats you consume should be predominantly monounsaturated and polyunsaturated fats.

When insulin is absent in the bloodstream (which occurs normally between meals if you do not snack), large quantities of fatty acids are released into the blood. This, in turn, causes the conversion of some fat into cholesterol. When this happens your cholesterol levels can rise dramatically. This high concentration of cholesterol, which can become extreme in cases of diabetes mellitus, may lead to the development of atherosclerosis, the clogging of the arteries.

Why Is Blood Sugar Regulation So Important?

A hormone that acts the opposite of insulin is glucagon. Glucagon is secreted by the pancreas when the concentration of blood sugar falls. Therefore, the role of glucagon is to increase blood glucose concentration. It does this by breaking down the glycogen stored in the liver into glucose and converting amino acids and fats into glucose.

There are three fundamental reasons why you should not allow your blood sugar concentration to rise too high:
1. Glucose causes great pressure in the fluid around cells, which can cause cellular dehydration if glucose levels get too high.
2. Excessive amounts of blood sugar can cause loss of glucose in the urine.
3. Since too much blood glucose can cause loss of glucose in the urine, pressure is created within the kidneys. This, in turn, can cause the depletion of essential body fluids and electrolytes.

To understand how various foods can stimulate rises in blood glucose, we need to discuss the glycemic index.

The Glycemic Index of Foods

According to Bill Kraemer and Jeff Volek of the Center for Sports Medicine at Penn State University, foods differ in the rate they are digested and converted into sugar. Sugar from digested foods moves into the bloodstream from the digestive system. Insulin is responsible for transporting sugar into the cells of the body for use as energy. This provides the basis for the glycemic index (GI) measurement of foods. The glycemic index indicates the rate at which foods are digested.

Foods that have a low GI promote a slow, steady rise in blood sugar as well as insulin after a meal. In contrast, foods that have a high GI result in a sharp increase in insulin, followed by a "crash" in the blood sugar concentration as insulin levels rise to move sugar into the cells of the body, which leaves blood sugar levels very low. I call this the sugar coma. Interestingly, the end result of ingesting high GI foods is increased appetite and fatigue, along with a greater tendency for the body to convert calories into body fat.

Variety and moderation are important concepts for optimal nutrition. A balance between high and low GI foods is a good strategy for designing a healthy, well-balanced, nutritional eating plan. From now on, you should strategically design your meals and snacks throughout the day, combining foods that are high in protein and moderate in fat with foods that have a high GI. When you eat high GI foods alone, your blood sugar levels rise rapidly, as does the ensuing insulin response. When you combine low GI foods (foods generally containing protein and fat) with high GI foods, the rise in glucose levels is not as fast so insulin does not store fat so readily. Combining low GI foods with high GI foods creates a buffer system to prevent fast rises in blood glucose levels.

Several factors determine the glycemic index:
• The type of sugar—fructose (fruit sugar) is lowest.
• Fiber content—soluble fiber is lower than insoluble.
• Protein and fat generally indicate a lower GI.
• Compact versus crumbly—compact foods tend to have a higher GI than crumbly foods (e.g., pasta has a higher GI than bread).
• Resistance to digestion (e.g., whole grain breads have a higher GI than breads made from refined flour).
• Amylose (sugar) versus amylopectin-starch (fiber)—sugary foods have a higher GI than fibrous and starchy foods.

The following chart shows the glycemic index of some common foods:*

Breads, Cereals, and Grains

All-Bran Cereal	50-80	Potatoes	>100
Barley	30-50	Pumpernickel	50-80
Bread, French	>100	Rice, Instant	>100
Bread, White	>100	Rice, Puffed	>100
Bread, Whole Wheat	80-100	Rice, White or Brown	80-100
Corn Flakes	>100	Rye, Whole Grain	30-50
Grapenuts	80-100	Spaghetti	50-80
Oat Bran	80-100	Wheat, Puffed	>100
Oatmeal (slow cook)	30-50	Wheat, Shredded	80-100
Pasta	50-80		

Vegetables

Beans, Baked	50-80	Corn	80-100
Beans, Kidney	30-50	Lentils	30-50
Beans, Lima	30-50	Peas	50-80
Beans, Navy	50-80	Peas, Black-eyed	30-50
Beans, Pinto	50-80	Peas, Chick	30-50

*Courtesy Bill Kraemer and Jeff Volek, Center for Sports Medicine at Penn State University

Beans, Soy	<30	Sweet Potatoes	30-50
Carrots	80-100	Tomato Soup	30-50

Fruits

Apples	30-50	Mangos	80-100
Apple Juice	30-50	Oranges	50-80
Applesauce	30-50	Orange Juice	50-80
Apricots	80-100	Papayas	80-100
Bananas	80-100	Peaches	30-50
Cherries	<30	Pears	30-50
Grapefruit	<30	Plums	<30
Grapes	30-50	Raisins	80-100

Dairy Products — *Snacks*

Ice Cream (low fat)	80-100	Candy Bars	30-50
Ice Cream (regular)	30-50	Corn Chips	80-100
Milk	30-50	Peanuts	<30
Yogurt	30-50	Rye Crisps	80-100

Sugars

Fructose	<30	Maltose	>100
Glucose	>100	Sucrose	50-80
Lactose	50-80		

Avoid Performance-Destroying Sugar Buzzes and Comas

Disregarding the consequences of highly refined sugar intake can weaken you when you need to be strongest. Sugar coma, as we use the term here, doesn't refer to actual unconsciousness. Rather, it means the energy-sapping and productivity-destroying sugar low that so often follows a sugar spike.

Sugar spike refers to the sudden jump in blood sugar caused by consuming too much simple sugar, particularly on an empty stomach. Simple-sugar foods—candy bars, cookies, jelly rolls, and some complex carbohydratres (carrots, rice, bananas) reach the bloodsteam quickly, where they can spike your blood sugar. The spike sends a hurry-up call to your pancreas to get things back to normal, which it does by releasing a flood of insulin. The insulin then pounds the sugar spike down, which puts you into a sugar coma, knocking your energy down and driving your productivity down. This release of insulin is also considered a major element in the body storing more fat.

It happens every day to millions of people in corporate America. After skipping breakfast, they swarm into the break room eager for a caffeine jolt and some sugary donuts or cookies. Their empty stomachs don't retain either the caffeine or the sugar for long, and within minutes they feel a surge of energy. That's the up, and it feels good. The down that strikes around lunchtime doesn't feel so good, and it isn't helped much by the usual corporate lunch—either a high-fat meal hurriedly scarfed down, or a high-fat, high caffeine (or alcohol) meal consumed at leisure. The worst productivity drop of the day usually hits in the midafternoon, when your natural circadian trough combines with an after-lunch sugar coma. Irritability, mistakes, and frustration often result.

We should consume only small amounts of simple sugar (cookies, candies) each day. A good rule is never to eat cookies, candy, or ice cream because you're hungry; eat them only for pleasure since they are low in nutrition but high in calories.

Many Europeans average only two servings of cookies or chocolates a day. That's very good. Most Americans have almost double that. We call them chocoholics.

When you tend toward hypoglycemia, you should take food with you wherever you go—the famous brown bag. Complex carbohydrates have a much slower release of blood sugar and are much better for you because your blood sugar isn't jumping up and down—your pancreas is functioning quietly, and all's well. Go for an apple, peach, or some other fruit instead of candy. The slight extra effort pays off in steadier blood-sugar levels and higher sustained energy and alertness.

Note the high amount of refined sugar in the Total Sugar column in the following table for every one of the candies, cookies, and other treats. By contrast, apples and other common fruits have no refined sugar (mostly fructose, which is slowly metabolized through the liver), no saturated fat, and fewer calories.

The first rule for not porking out at break time is to avoid getting to the break room in a ravenous state of mind. In other words, make your previous meal large enough to carry you to break time in comfort. All too often people charge into the

break room too hungry to care what they eat. The second rule is
to select a low-fat snack.

Snack	Calories	Total Carbohydrates	Complex Carbohydrates	Total Sugar	Total Fat
2 oz. M&M's chocolate	270	38.7g	4.04g	32.9g	12.5g
2 oz. M&M's peanut	281	33.5g	5.24g	26.6g	15.3g
2 oz. Licorice	208	52.8g	0.1g	52.7g	0.3g
2 oz. Snickers	258	34.2g	5.8g	26.9g	12.7g
2 oz. Mars	265	35.6g	1.9g	32.7g	13g
2 oz. Angel Food Cake	147	32.7g	6.1g	26.5g	0.5g
2 oz. Choc. Cupcake	208	30.9g	1.7g	29.2g	9.3g
2 oz. Hard Candy	212	55.6g	0.6g	55.0g	0g
2 oz. Butter Cookie	265	39.0g	18.7g	17.9g	10.7g
2 oz. Apple Pie	134	19.3g	10.6g	7.8g	6.25g

What a Difference a Snack Makes

Since snacks should only be a small part of your diet, you
may be inclined to ignore Anti-Dieting principles when grabbing
a quick snack. Aside from the fact that you can load a lot of extra
calories and fat into your average intake that way, you can also
destroy your performance at a crucial time. Maybe you'll blow a
presentation, flub an important negotiation, or wonder why you
didn't play a more decisive role in a staff meeting.

The world will never know how many millions of business
situations get botched because someone's blood sugar dropped
below the base line, and his or her brain stuttered, misfired, and
made mistakes. When something like this happens in business,
the pressure of the moment and whatever disappointment and
humiliation were involved tend to mask the physiological reasons why the failure occurred. People tend to blame themselves
and hack away at their self-esteem rather than look for a simple physical explanation.

I suspect that the phenomenon of sudden blood sugar
troughing occurs constantly in many human activities. It certainly does in the sports world, where I happened to witness a
dramatic instance at the U.S. Open in the 1990s.

Boris Becker, the great German tennis star, was down two
sets to one against Brad Gilbert, an always dangerous American
opponent. Early in the fourth set, Becker wanted something to
eat, and his manager quickly brought him a candy bar.

I watched Becker eat the candy bar on a changeover, and the results were quite interesting. Although Becker's serving percentages didn't change much from what they had been in the previous sets, he did go on to win the fourth set and tie the match at two sets all. The fifth set would decide the match.

Now, we are talking about the latter stages of an important match at a grand slam event between two highly ranked players. Up for grabs: massive amounts of prestige and important money. Bear in mind that Boris Becker was a big, strong, and very fit athlete in his 20s. You wouldn't think he would fade physically—but he did! In the final set, Becker's serving percentages dropped, his unforced errors soared, and he lost. Could it be that the "buzz" (the sugar spike) he got from eating the candy bar did not significantly affect his game, but that the following sugar coma nailed him? My guess is, "Yes!"

Some research says that simple sugar intake has little or no effect on large muscle groups in sports like running or cycling. However, tennis is also a fine muscle-control sport where thoughts and small movements may make the difference. Some theories suggest that the same is true for emotional control and the ability to access the Ideal Performance State in business and life.

Unless you're convinced you have a far greater resistance to sugar spikes and comas than three-time Wimbledon champion Boris Becker, avoid eating a high-sugar snack or candy before facing an important challenge. Eating an apple instead could save your day!

Eat a variety of foods. Eat five or six small meals a day. Eat large meals only on very special occasions. Eat fresh food whenever you can. Eat red meat no more than twice a week. Avoid egg yolks. Enjoying one alcoholic drink a day won't hurt you, but more will. Eat baked or grilled fresh fish two or three times a week and shellfish no more than once a week. Prefer bottled water to chlorinated city water. Eat one third more carbohydrates than protein.

Strategic Snacking All Day Long

About 87 percent of the executives who attend my seminar report that they eat three meals or less in one day, and about 13 percent eat four or five meals a day. A few people report that they regularly have only one meal a day.

From two important standpoints, that's not smart at all: (1) They have difficulty maintaining effective levels of blood sugar throughout the day, and (2) they are training their bodies to store fat. One-meal eaters can vastly improve their performance by reorganizing their daily routines so that they eat five small meals a day instead of one large one. Such a drastic change in eating habits should be spread out over several days.

Make time for a small, nutritious breakfast followed by small meals (like an apple) every two hours or so throughout the day. Research and experience proves that this deserves high priority. I call it *strategic snacking,* and it's the heart of Anti-Dieting. When this health and performance-building pattern culminates with a small early dinner, you're all set for a good night's rest.

For breakfast, I typically have cereal and low-fat milk. About 90 minutes later I'll eat an apple. Around 11:30 I'll probably have an orange. So I eat just little bits of food all morning. I strongly recommend it to you because it keeps your metabolism up.

If, instead of strategic snacking, you eat three big meals a day, your blood sugar goes up and down. Avoiding wide swings in blood sugar is especially important for corporate executives because the brain works on oxygen and glucose. With low glucose you're not as good cognitively because glucose is "thought fuel." When that tank is low, your thinking processes work slower, some of your cylinders might not fire, and you're likely to make mistakes.

You can eat an apple (about 100 calories) midmorning to stabilize your blood sugar. The important thing is to avoid slipping into performance-destroying blood sugar troughs.

To avoid the troughs, you may have to change some habits. Get away from having a big breakfast and then a big snack. You don't want to eat big, big, big, and then snack, snack, snack.

Then in a year when you've gained weight you'll call me to say you don't like my program!

You should eat a small breakfast, small snack, small lunch. When do you have your big meal of the day? Never, except when you're at Grandma Millie's for Thanksgiving or Christmas. Even then you don't have to stuff your cheeks. Train Grandma Millie away from her notion that you need second helpings of all her myriad dishes. If necessary, be a little firm about it.

If you're serious about reaching high velocity toward attaining your maximum potential, you never overeat, never have a huge meal. Your nourishment rhythm is a small-to-moderate meal, then a snack; a small-to-moderate meal, then another snack. We strongly recommend this rhythm to stabilize your blood sugar throughout your day. After a few weeks on this regimen, you'll be amazed at how well, and how alert, you feel.

Anything under 200 calories is a snack; a small meal is 200 to 350 calories; 500 calories is a moderate meal; over 750 calories is a big meal.

These food strategies will also help you to discover your ultimate potential and create the physical, mental, and emotional toughness required to reach maximum velocity in your life.

Do you know how the military turns young recruits into tough soldiers? They literally teach them to be good actors, to look alert, energetic, and unafraid regardless of how they feel. You must do the same as a Corporate Athlete. Good nutrition helps.

Train Your Fat Cells Right by Eating Often

Skipping meals and fasting for extended periods train your body to store fat against the next shortage of food. Here's how it works: When you fast, lipogenesis enzymes, already programmed to absorb fat, have nothing to work on. The body says, "I'm starving, so I must protect myself to survive. I'll store fat like crazy when I can." As a result they create more enzymes, which create more fat when food becomes available. The quickest way to build a potbelly is to eat only one meal a day because you keep your body on famine alert.

If weight loss is your aim, minimize the lipogenesis

enzyme action by never allowing yourself to get hungry. Take care to always have a good breakfast, enjoy a low-fat mid-morning snack, and eat a nutritious lunch. Then, have a nonfat snack in midafternoon so you don't go to the dinner table feeling ravenous. The body now says, "What, more food already? I'll boost my metabolism to get rid of it." The opposite course—skipping breakfast, skimping on lunch, and eating heavy in the evening—works against weight loss.

"Eating frequent, smaller meals throughout the day actually revs up your metabolic rate," writes Kim Galeaz, a registered dietitian who is also associated with the American Dietetic Association. What happens is simple: Food digestion takes energy, and its thermic effect causes the body to dissipate heat, a process that burns calories and fat. "The effect lasts about five hours," says David Levitsky, a professor of nutrition and psychology at Cornell University. "If you eat infrequently, there's clearly a metabolic slowdown." Eating five small meals a day can keep your metabolism rate at a high, fat-burning rate all day long.

Winning the Fight Against Your Body's Fear of Famine

Winning the fight against your body's fear of famine (without dying in the process via *anorexia nervosa*) is possible if your goal is to improve your ratio of fat to lean body mass. Here are four tactics to make this easier:

1. Keep your caloric intake consistent from day to day. Avoid repeatedly making wide swings in your daily caloric intake. If your reducing plan calls for 2,000 calories a day, work at staying as close to that number as you can. Especially avoid deliberate wide swings—eating, for example, 2,800 calories one day and 1,500 the next "to make up for it." How does the body react to wide swings? First, it gleefully stores fat on the 2,800 calorie day, and then on the 1,500 calorie day it slows its metabolism so it won't have to use its reserves of fat to continue normal functions. Then, with the famine-avoidance training you've just given it, your body can probably manage to continue storing a little fat when you return to your normal reducing diet of 2,000 calories a day. This explanation simplifies a very complex process, but the essential message is accurate: Constant changes in the volume of food intake work against weight loss; consistency in the amount of food intake makes a reducing plan more effective.

2. *Eat several small meals a day.* Four to six small meals instead of two or three large ones. By never getting too hungry, you dull your body's fear of famine and keep your metabolism at a high, fat-burning level.

3. *Build variety into your consistent diet.* The calorie total is the important element to maintain at a consistent level. Vary the types and mix of carbohydrates, protein, and fat as necessary.

4. *Adjust your diet slowly.* Change your breakfast one week, your midmorning snack the next, then your lunch, and so on until you are fully on the plan. If you're not changing foods, but rather the quantities, bring what you're eating into line with your reducing plan by cutting out no more than one serving a day.

Chapter 4

STRATEGIES FOR EATING AND DRINKING YOUR WAY TO HIGHER VELOCITY AND HAPPINESS

"An army marches on its stomach."
—Napoleon Bonaparte

More and more people are coming to this realization: Eating right is not only a major challenge, it is an ongoing battle of enormous importance in achieving success. There are two parts to this matter: the negative one of eliminating the energy-sapping handicap of carrying extra weight, and the positive one of gaining the high-performance benefits conferred by eating right and being fit.

I'm going to give you strategies not only for discovering your Ideal Performance State (IPS), but also for accessing it whenever you desire. In this chapter, I'll discuss the physical, mental, and emotional toughening required to reach maximum velocity in your life through achieving and maintaining IPS when you need it. Good nutrition is an essential precondition. Your engine can't reach full power if it's not well-fueled.

The brain works on two things: oxygen and glucose. Carbohydrates ensure that the nerve system and the brain are functioning properly.

Carbohydrates Versus Proteins

Nutritional thinking is beginning to swing away from the 65 percent complex carbohydrates, 15 percent protein, and 20 percent fat formula widely accepted in the 1980s. Although that formula was once regarded as "the ideal we're shooting for in sport recovery," according to William Kraemer of Pennsylvania State University, "it begins to be a demanding challenge to eat that way."

With formulas running all over the place (some recommending as high as 57 percent protein) it becomes difficult to settle on what's best for your individual situation. With the high-protein diets, the high-fat diets, and the high-carbohydrate diets, you have a variety of nutritional camps out there pushing their particular approaches. Under the appropriate circumstances and for the right people, they might all work, but how they affect performance and recovery is just beginning to be known.

As Kraemer points out, even some endurance runners, who know they should be eating 65 percent carbohydrates, don't actually eat that way all the time. Most of them maintain a level of about 50 percent, and then during certain brief loading periods before a race, they bring it up to around 65 percent.

The Effects of Carbohydrates

Are carbohydrates unnecessary, as some protein enthusiasts claim? Kraemer says it's like saying a strong forehand isn't necessary in tennis. A player who hits all aces and backhands and only a few forehands can do well with a weak forehand. The body is an amazing machine: In six to eight weeks it can adapt to whatever diet you force it to use.

Some people, eating 65 percent carbohydrates, become water-sensitive. They start to have problems because more carbohydrates drag more water into their cells. This, in addition to the insulin response to the rise in glucose, can also cause an increase in body fat. Sometimes people even gain weight on 65 percent carbohydrates, but in reality they're only getting more thoroughly hydrated.

On the other hand, a high-protein diet may bring a lot of fat with it and can cause calcium depletion in your body. Anyone adopting such a diet needs to remain alert to the dangers involved in consuming large amounts of fat—including rapid weight gain, high cholesterol levels, and heart disease.

The Food-Mood Connection

The latest research into the food-mood connection has been called "tantalizing, but inconsistent and incomplete." In other words, we may be close to knowing exactly how we can powerfully influence—or even control—how we feel through what, how much, and when we eat. Or maybe not. This is not far-fetched. Many people have long known how certain eating or imbibing behaviors affect them. Here are three examples:

1. Someone eats a big meal on his day off and says, "I'm going to watch the football game," but before the first quarter ends, he's sound asleep.

2. Working late to prepare for an especially heavy day makes a sales manager eat late. More drinks than she really needs accompany the late dinner. After the alarm pounds her awake the next morning, she's in no mood for breakfast, and she begins her especially heavy workday in a sugar coma—hung over, tired, and depressed. As a result she fails to perform at her highest potential.

3. For breakfast, a hungry person eats a stack of syrup-soaked pancakes washed down with coffee—heading for the old caffeine jolt, plus diuretic action with a sugar spike on the way. He gets the jolt after an hour and feels alert but dry-mouthed, hyper, and a bit shaky. Two hours later his alertness fades into weariness. He's drinking a lot of water without fully slaking his thirst, and he feels like he's gone four rounds with a hard puncher.

Yes, it is true we can influence our mood and performance potential by what, when, and how much we eat and drink. But, regrettably, what we learn by trial and error tends toward how to avoid damage to our performance potential rather than toward how to enhance it.

Several studies show that meals rich in carbohydrates and low in protein have a mild sedative effect. The largest study, conducted by Harvard University and other institutions, discovered that women felt sleepier, and men more relaxed, after eating a carbohydrate-rich meal as compared to one rich in protein.

Research also suggests that frequent small meals sustain

alertness far better than fewer and heavier meals. In particular, a heavy lunch has been shown to increase errors on tasks requiring close attention, while a light lunch reduces them. A nutritious late-afternoon snack also decreases errors.

How Your Brain Uses Food

The brain synthesizes dopamine, norepinephrine, and serotonin from amino acids. Amino acids are the building blocks of protein; protein is the building block of life. Two of these amino acids—tyrosine and tryptophan—are critical to maintaining the Ideal Performance State.

Tyrosine comes from protein; tryptophan comes mainly from carbohydrates. Eating any form of protein, alone or in combination with other foods, makes tyrosine available to the brain. The brain synthesizes dopamine and norepinephrine from tyrosine.

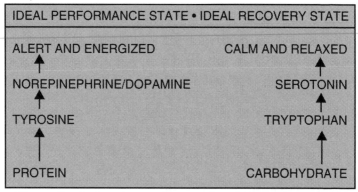

If your brain is using up its supply of dopamine and norepinephrine, more is synthesized. If your brain still has plenty, it will not make more.

This leads us to a vital point about mood food: The barrier or pathway across the membrane surrounding the brain provides only limited access to the amino acids generated by food consumption. The amino acids don't go right in just because they are there. It's much like a freeway on-ramp controlled by a signal during rush hour. Only so much can get through.

For this discussion, let's assume your brain has low amounts of Ideal Recovery State hormones—serotonin. When you eat protein and carbohydrates together, tyrosine and tryptophan are released, but because it is the smaller of the two amino acids, tryptophan just gets crowded out. The only way to get tryptophan into the brain is to eat carbohydrates alone—candy, fruit, salad, or pasta. This causes a release of insulin from the pancreas to regulate blood sugar. All other amino acids then go to work on other cellular activities in the body's systems: skeletal, digestive, circulatory, muscular, nervous. Now there's more tryptophan available in the blood, and voilà, it's off to the brain.

Eaten by themselves, carbohydrates stimulate the production of serotonin, the calming hormone. When carbohydrates are eaten in combination with protein, the protein prevents the production of serotonin and stimulates the development of the chemicals dopamine and norepinephrine.

How much does it take to do the trick? Four ounces of animal protein will increase tyrosine in the blood and thus increase IPS hormones—dopamine and norepinephrine.

One and a half ounces of fruit, salad, sweets, or starch will increase tryptophan levels and IRS hormones in the blood. (Overweight people or women who are menstruating may need two and a half ounces.)

But doubling your protein intake won't make you twice as alert, and doubling your carbohydrate intake won't make you twice as calm. Don't get caught up in the "more is better" syndrome—it doesn't work.

Avoiding Simple Sugars

Try to avoid refined carbohydrates. A refined carbohydrate is a food that has been processed until it has virtually no nutrients left. For example, a single slice of white bread is about 65 calories— slightly more than whole wheat—but it supplies only a fourth as much fiber and almost no vitamins or minerals—in two words: no nutrition. Although white bread will create glycogen, it's a nutritionally non-dense food when compared with vegetables and fresh fruits, which have fewer calories but are very high in nutrition.

We should consume small amounts of simple sugars each day. In my experience, only 23 percent of corporate executives have two or fewer servings of sugar a day—as in cookies, chocolates, or sugar spooned into coffee. Most of my other audiences are more on the chocoholic side, averaging well over two servings of sugar a day. This can have an immediate effect on performance.

A study performed ten years ago showed a male office worker who consumed only a large chocolate candy bar at lunch. About 30 minutes later, when his blood sugar had spiked, his phone rang:

"Hello? No problem, I'll get on that right away. Thank you for calling. Bye."

About 40 minutes after that, his body's response to the sugar spike hit in the form of a massive insulin release from his pancreas. The insulin drove his blood sugar level below where it had been before he ate the candy bar, putting him in a sugar coma. Then the phone rang again; it was someone with the same problem as the previous caller.

Now, the office worker couldn't perform at the level of only 40 minutes earlier; he answered the phone without enthusiasm and mumbled, "Hello, yes. Uh, that's a tough one. Hold on. I'll have to transfer you to someone else."

If he had snacked on an apple instead of the candy bar, his energy level would have remained high. His blood sugar would have risen slowly and not spiked. But instead, his blood sugar was driven below the level necessary to sustain alertness and energy because the insulin rushed to counter the sugar spike.

Fueling with Fiber

You should consume moderate to high amounts of fiber every day. Corporate America is fast becoming very good about this. Nearly half of the executives who atttend my corporate conferences report intentionally eating food that is high in fiber. That's much greater than among some of the other audiences I work with.

At the other end of the spectrum, some people get so carried away with fiber that they take fiber supplements. You do not need them. I align my own thoughts to those of Bill Cosby: He says, "Fiber? It just helps move things along!"

Fiber can be water soluble or water insoluble. Neither kind provides energy, but both have other important functions.

Insoluble fiber is nondigestible and acts like a sponge, absorbing water to help waste products pass easily and swiftly through the colon. It is the best cure or prevention for constipation. Many studies have confirmed that a high-fiber diet reduces the incidence of colon cancer, and a low-fiber diet has the opposite effect.

If you eat a diet that's 50 percent carbohydrates you will get enough fiber. Fruits and whole-grain foods are high in fiber. Apple skins and the chaff of grain have fiber. Insoluble fiber is found in the rind of some fruits—in the membrane of oranges, for example.

Water-soluble fiber, found in oat bran, barley, and fruit pectin, helps reduce cholesterol levels, primarily by reducing low-density lipoproteins (LDL—the "bad" cholesterol). However, researchers debate exactly how much water-soluble fiber is required to achieve this effect, and many suggest that the benefit comes as much from the reduction in fat consumption that occurs in a high-fiber diet as from the action of the fiber itself. Until this is clarified the best course is just to eat a high-fiber diet.

As for what research says about fiber intake, some studies also suggest that insoluble fiber helps control diabetes by improving your control of blood sugar. Future research may also confirm current theories that a high-fiber diet reduces the risk of breast cancer. Eating high-fiber foods also helps reduce obesity because these foods take longer to chew and provide a filled-up feeling without adding many calories.

To guarantee that your fiber intake is adequate, eat a variety of foods. Whenever you have a choice, buy or order the least-processed alternative. Raw fruits, vegetables and grains are best.

Avoid getting all your fiber at one sitting because this can have unpleasant side effects. Instead, try to eat foods that are high in both kinds of fiber at every meal. A high-fiber diet increases your need for water, so be sure to accompany it with a high fluid intake.

Boost Your Productivity with Fresh Produce

Why would you want to eat more bananas and broccoli when what you would really like is a thick steak and a baked potato smothered in butter and sour cream? For three reasons:

- Eating enough fruits and vegetables helps protect you against a long list of degenerative and chronic diseases headed by coronary heart disease and many kinds of cancer.
- Eating a heavy steak and fat-added baked potato does exactly the opposite by moving you closer to the same list of killer diseases.
- Eating five to seven servings of fruits and vegetables a day is essential to reaching and sustaining your maximum career potential and personal energy level.

If you now eat very few fresh fruits and vegetables a day, increase your consumption of them slowly. Add no more than a serving a week. Always give your body time to adjust.

Before you tense up at the thought of downing seven servings of fruit and vegetables every day, remember that a serving is any of the following:

- One cup of raw leafy vegetables.
- One half cup of cooked vegetables.
- One quarter cup of dried fruit.
- One medium-size piece of fruit: an apple, banana, pear, or peach; one third of a cantaloupe; one half of a grapefruit; a half-moon shaped piece of watermelon one inch thick; or one half cup of berries.
- One medium-size vegetable: a full-size carrot or one or two small stalks of celery.

Obviously, you shouldn't get too precise when dealing with fruits and vegetables, so look on these definitions of servings as rough guidelines.

Your absolute minimum for improved performance is five servings of fruit and vegetables every day—for maximum performance and velocity, seven servings. Every day. Eat them in combination with an otherwise well-balanced nutrition and exercise program, featuring quality proteins and other low-fat foods. You'll feel more alert, have more stamina, sleep better, and handle stress more easily. Since this will provide ample fiber, you'll also be able to throw your laxatives away.

I emphasize a well-balanced nutrition and exercise program because some people think, "If seven servings of fruit and vegetables a day will boost my output, fourteen a day will give me phenomenal performance." Please don't try it. Within days you'll have a bad case of diarrhea, and you'll hate the sight of fruit so much you'll drop back to a diet dangerously low in fresh produce and be worse off than before. Sustained benefit—what Anti-Dieting calls for—comes from eating an adequate amount of fruits and vegetables plus all the proteins and other essentials a high-performance body requires.

25 Ways to Eat More Fruits and Vegetables

You may think that consuming seven servings of fruit and vegetables every day will be quite a departure from your present way of eating, but let's look at 25 ways you can boost your productivity with fresh produce.

For Breakfast:
1. Prepare your pancakes or waffles with sliced apples or berries in the batter. Top them off with more fruit.
2. Make a sandwich of your breakfast toast and whatever fruits sound appealing: blueberries, strawberries, raspberries, or apples and cinnamon.
3. Add sliced bananas, peaches, apples, raisins, berries, prunes, or any other fruit to your hot or cold cereal. It only takes one quarter of a cup of dried fruit such as apricots, dates, or a half cup of berries to make a serving.
4. Whip up a vegetable omelet with Eggbeaters or egg whites only. Practically any vegetable can be an ingredient in a vegetable omelet, but some of the most popular are chopped onions, peppers, tomatoes, mushrooms, broccoli, and zucchini.

For Morning Snacks:
5. If you're on the run, apples, raisins, bagels, or nuts will make a convenient snack capable of regulating your blood sugar level to keep your energy output high. Almost any other tasty fruit will have the same effect.

For Lunch:
6. Use romaine lettuce, chicory, or spinach as a bed for your salad; a cup of any of them makes a serving. They're all

far more nutritious than the more popular iceberg lettuce. Add another cup of any combination of chopped carrots, celery, broccoli, cucumber, mushrooms, tomatoes, or peppers, and your salad counts as two servings toward your goal of seven. Add sliced oranges or pineapple on top and you've hit three servings.

7. Have a bowl of hearty vegetable soup. If you can control how it's made, have it made thick so a cup of it amounts to a half cup of vegetables. A half cup of cooked vegetables is a full serving.

8. Enjoy a baked potato without loading it up with fat from butter, cheese, and sour cream. If you've always soaked the potato with the high-fat additives, you may want to cut back gradually: Use a little less butter or sour cream each time. You can also experiment with low-fat alternatives: Molly McButter, Butter Buds, sliced green onions, chives, soy sauce, nonfat yogurt, or sour cream.

The baked potato with skin, without additives, delivers only 225 calories: 51 grams of carbohydrate, 4.7 grams of protein, and a mere 0.2 of a gram of fat. Adding 2 tablespoons of butter piles on an additional 203 calories and 23 grams of fat. Slap on just 2 tablespoons of sour cream and you've added another 174 calories and 22 grams of fat. It makes a total of 45 grams of fat and 377 calories added to the almost fat-free potato.

Instead of the baked russet potato you may be loading up with calorie-heavy and fat-laden condiments, you might try sweet or redskin potatoes. They don't need additives to make them taste great.

9. Add a full serving of fruit to a yogurt dessert by adding berries or a sliced banana or peach.

10. If you choose a pasta entree or a rice salad, add interest to these dishes with tomatoes, broccoli, carrots, cucumber, peppers, or mushrooms.

11. Have your sandwich stuffed with bean sprouts, shredded carrots, or tomatoes. Add a few slices of apple or pear to your meal.

12. To move one serving closer to your goal of seven, pick

up a peach, pear, sliced pineapple, or some grapes. Many salad bars offer them.

For Afternoon Snacks

13. Keep bite-size pieces of fruit on hand for snacks: Apricots, dates, and strawberries are naturally bite-size. Sliced kiwi, mangos, and melon are great if they're around.

14. Keep bite-size vegetables on hand: Carrots, celery, broccoli, and cauliflower can be purchased in bite-size pieces.

For Dinner:

15. We have a curious idea in the States: Grapefruit is strictly for breakfast. But a half grapefruit makes a wonderful appetizer before any meal.

16. Speaking of wonderful appetizers, a small fruit salad, a cup of cold fruit on a hot day, or a dish of sliced strawberries will deliver a pleasant wake-up call to your taste buds.

17. Explore the wide variety of vegetable appetizers: Veggie sticks with a low-fat or nonfat yogurt dip, eggplant with ricotta, or fricasseed mushrooms are only a few of the possibilities.

18. Carrot and celery sticks in a bowl of ice have long been a staple on many tables. Expand this excellent idea to include chopped cauliflower, green beans, summer squash, broccoli, and peppers.

19. Corn cut off the cob is great for thickening soups or gravies.

20. Boost the nutritional value of stews and casseroles with extra vegetables.

21. Replace cheese dip with salsa. If your reaction is, "Yuck," you may be hooked on high-fat foods to a dangerous degree. Remember: You can train yourself to prefer fat-free salsa over fat-heavy cheese dip. Training yourself to prefer low-fat or fat-free foods is the key to solving the excessive fat-storage problem.

22. Tasty vegetables should accompany your dinner entree. Glazed carrots, wild or brown rice, broccoli, and sweet corn are just a few of your choices.

For Dessert:

23. Nutritionally speaking, fruit is an ideal dessert at dinner-time because it won't interfere with sleep. For a tasty finale to a nutritious meal, choose a bowl of cherries or strawberries, or a baked apple (one not drowned in sugar).

24. If your vice in the evening is ice cream, try low-fat or fat-free frozen yogurt, ice cream, or ice milk. Just be sure to watch for high sugar content. Top your treat off with a serving of berries or sliced peaches.

25. Avoid desserts such as peach cobblers and sugary apple pies because they bury the fruit in sugar. Instead, top off a slice of angel food cake with cherries, berries, or fresh peaches.

Avoid the Lowfat Food Trap

Wouldn't it be great if we could lose weight just by cutting all fat out of our diets? This wonderfully simple approach sounds terrific until you discover it doesn't work. If you consume more calories than you burn, you'll gain weight. Don't be fooled by misleading labels: "fat-free" doughnuts and cookies are loaded with calories, mostly from simple sugars.

Powering with Protein

The popular concept of the high-protein power lunch has faded into folk myth, along with yesteryear's steak-and-eggs training tables. The plain truth is that if you need quick energy, you must find it in carbohydrates—not meat, fish, eggs, and other high-protein foods. Yet protein and fat, though often unpopular with many people, are an essential part of everyone's diet. In corporate America, however, the problem can more likely be too much protein rather than too little. For maximum performance, Corporate Athletes should limit their protein intake to about one fourth to one third of their food consumption.

Nutritionists are zeroing in on how much protein people need to perform at their highest levels. Bear this in mind: Just eating more protein alone doesn't build muscle—your best bet is resistance training.

The more active you are, the more protein you need (within limits). Here is a quick readout of how much net protein you should be eating for maximum productivity and energy:

Sedentary:	.4 grams per pound of body weight
Moderately Active:	.6 grams per pound of body weight
Very Active:	.8 grams per pound of body weight

Thus, a 200-pound active male athlete requires 160 grams of net protein daily; a 110-pound sedentary female requires only 40 grams of net protein daily.

What is meant by "net" protein? The animal sources of protein—seafood and meat—are about 40 percent fat, so our 200-pound active athlete needs to eat the equivalent of a 9.5 ounce steak each day.

To obtain the proper net protein amounts suggested, eat the following gross amounts of protein:

Sedentary: for each pound of body weight, eat .66 grams of fish or meat. (Multiply your weight in pounds by .66 grams.) To convert the resulting allowance from grams to ounces, divide by 28. Thus, a 130-pound sedentary person should consume about 3 ounces of fish or meat daily.

Moderately Active: 1 gram of fish or meat per pound of body weight. This works out to a little more than 5 ounces of seafood or meat a day for a 150-pound moderately active person.

Very Active: 1.33 grams of fish or meat per pound of body weight. This is about 10 ounces of seafood or steak daily for a 200-pound person who is very active physically.

You may prefer to consume all or part of your daily protein requirement in vegetable form.

Protein—If You Prefer to Eat Meatless

Can you imagine prehistoric humans worrying about food combinations as they foraged through the grasslands? They ate what and when they could. And if you eat sensibly, you can, too. Contrary to what we used to hear, it's not necessary to combine grains and legumes in the same meal to acquire useable protein. Eat common foods such as whole-grain breads,

potatoes, and corn to meet your daily requirement for protein.
Fruit is a poor source of protein, as are alcohol, sugar, and fat.
Here are some excellent vegetable sources of protein:

One cup servings: *Protein grams*
    Barley 5
    Beans, black 15.2
    Beans, kidney 15
    Beans, lima 14.7
    Beans, pinto 14
    Beans, white 17.5
    Broccoli 6
    Corn 6
    Lentils 18
    Spinach 6
    Rice, brown 5
    Rice, white 4
    Spaghetti 5
Single vegetable servings:
    Potato (including skin) 5
    Sweet Potato (including skin) 1.7
Other non-meat sources of protein:
    Skim Milk (8 oz. glass) 6
Two ounce servings:
    Almonds 10
    Macadamia Nuts 4
    Peanuts 13
    Pecans 4
    Walnuts 12

15 Foods and Food Groups that Help You Slim Down

The following foods aren't magic bullets, but choosing
these 15 foods instead of the higher-fat items they replace will
make a considerable difference over time.

Veal. It's readily available, relatively inexpensive, and lowfat.
Roasted veal sirloin with the fat trimmed off is only 33 percent
fat—10 percent lower in fat than the best beef. But remember,
with veal, as with all foods, you can lose the low-fat advantage in

the cooking, such as when it's breaded and fried in oil.

Exotic Meats. These may be hard to find, but they're often worth the trouble from the low-fat nutritional standpoint. Many mountain restaurants offer these delicacies. The exotic low-fat meats include venison and buffalo (American bison). Roasted venison is only 18 percent fat; bison is even lower—a mere 15 percent. No wonder our native Americans were so healthy when buffalo was an important part of their diet.

On the other hand, one of the fattest meats you can find is prime rib; when roasted it's a whopping, artery-clogging 62 percent fat! Roasted filet mignon of beef, trimmed, is 43 percent fat.

Poultry. Skinless chicken and turkey are lower in fat than beef or pork. However, not all poultry is lower in fat content than beef. Here are the numbers:

Chicken Breast (skinless) . . . . .19 percent fat
Duck (skinless, roasted) . . . . .19 percent fat
Goose (skinless, roasted) . . . . .48 percent fat
Quail (skinless, roasted) . . . . .22 percent fat
Squab Pigeon (skinless, raw) . . . . . .48 percent fat
Turkey Breast (skinless, roasted) . . .13 percent fat

Fish and Seafood. Many varieties of fish are far lower in fat than red meat, especially trout, cod, and snapper. Swordfish is the most likely to have a toxically high mercury content; cod the least so. Salmon, although rather fatty, contains oils (the omega fatty acids) that tend to increase the best factor in cholesterol, high-density lipoproteins (HDLs).

With any fish, as with red meat, how the food is prepared has a great deal to do with how much fat a forkful contains. Baking or broiling are the two best methods of minimizing fat; frying in batter and grease, or sautéing in butter boost the fat content considerably.

Cod (baked filet) . . . . 7 percent fat
Crab Legs, Alaskan King (steamed)   14 percent fat
Crayfish . . . . .13 percent fat
Lobster Tail (baked) . . . . .23 percent fat
Salmon, Atlantic (baked filet) . . . . . .40 percent fat
Salmon, Coho (steamed) . . . . .37 percent fat
Scallops (steamed) . . . . .27 percent fat

Shrimp (large, steamed) . . . . .10 percent fat
Shrimp (medium, baked) . . . . .29 percent fat
Snapper (baked filet) . . . . .12 percent fat
Swordfish (baked) . . . . .29 percent fat
Trout, Rainbow (baked filet) . . . . . .35 percent fat

High-Fiber Cereals. High-fiber cereals deliver a pleasant, filled-up feeling with fewer calories by providing bulk. According to one recent study, people who start the day with a high fiber cereal consume fewer calories during mid-morning snacks. Check the labels for high-fiber and low sugar, and use skim milk instead of whole milk. For an extra nutrition boost, add a fresh fruit topping.

Bagels. The cinnamon-raisin varieties are particularly good because they're sweet enough to keep you from piling on a fattening spread. Choose the small or medium-size bagels: The big ones run up your calorie count. If you absolutely must spread something on your bagel, try a teaspoon of low-sugar jam preserves.

Sweet Potatoes. Unlike russet potatoes, sweet potatoes don't beg for butter and sour cream to liven them up, although many people appreciate the delicate flavors of the naked russet. If you haven't reached this point yet, go for the naturally rich taste of the sweet potato.

Low-Fat (or Nonfat) Cream Cheese. The five grams of fat per spoonful of regular cream cheese have been reduced to three in the low-fat cream cheeses widely available at this writing. That's a 40-percent reduction in fat! Cream cheese lovers can train themselves to prefer the low-fat variety. However, today there are even fat-free varieties of cream cheese. If their taste doesn't appeal today, recheck every six months because the food industry is making rapid progress at improving fat-free taste.

Make a goal of training your taste buds to enjoy the fat-free version of cream cheese, a food whose flavor will gradually improve as time passes and consumer pressure increases. Start your move in this healthy direction by getting used to the low-fat kind.

Flavored Mineral Waters and Seltzers. Check the labels, but most flavored mineral waters and seltzers have far less sugar and calories than the usual soft drinks. The nonflavored varieties have no sugar or calories at all, but you may find them less than exciting. As the studies indicate, many people mistake thirst for hunger and eat when a drink of flavored water, or even plain water, would satisfy them.

Fresh Fruits. When you sit down to relax after a hard day, are you tempted to munch on chips or cookies? Try grapes instead; they're low in fat and tasty, especially when chilled. The time it takes to peel an orange can be a valuable weight-loss factor: It simply gives you time to read your body's messages. Eating the orange instead of drinking its juice gives you more fiber in a snack of only about 70 calories. A cup of orange juice has almost twice as much.

Salsa. Salsa is a terrific substitute for the goo and grease of mayonnaise on sandwiches, and as a marinade on fish or chicken. However, not all salsas are uniformly low calorie or low-fat. Some are oil-based. Check the label or ask your server if the salsa contains oil.

Air-Popped Popcorn. Four cups of air-popped popcorn contain only 100 calories and one gram of fat. The same amount of potato chips dumps nearly 600 calories and 40 grams of fat into your system. Air-popped is the key qualification. Many theaters now pop popcorn in healthier ways than they did in the 1980s. Most have banished the grease, lard, and tropical oils they once used, but it's still worth checking.

Pretzels. The low-fat, low-sodium brands are among the healthiest and most convenient snacks you can find.

Candy Bars. Almost everyone eating mostly low-fat, low-sugar foods is tempted to binge now and then. Set your safety valve well below the point of binge explosion; you don't have to be a fanatic to lose weight. In fact, fanaticism about fat can be life-threatening, as in anorexia.

Buying an individually packaged candy bar now and then to meet sweet tooth needs is a safer choice than ice cream, cakes, or packaged cookies. And polishing off a candy bar is aesthetically and emotionally more satisfying than scooping out just one serving of ice cream and leaving the rest of the gallon in the freezer, where it exerts a constant temptation to binge. The same holds true of the remaining cake or cookies.

Watch Low-Fat Foods

Be careful: Because of the idea that low-fat means "eat more," you can eat too much of the low-fat or nonfat foods. If you consume enough calories, your body will make and store fat no matter how little dietary fat you eat. Don't gorge. Too much food turns into too much fat.

Chapter 5

EATING RIGHT WHEN YOU'RE MOVING FAST

*"The larger your muscles, the more fat you
can burn immediately after exercise
and when your body is resting."*
—Fred Surgent

Most of the time, you're too busy for leisurely meals. For some of you, your nutrition comes from fast-food outlets and airplane meals. Even when you're not traveling, you and your spouse eat out almost every night.

Eating Healthier in the Fast-Fat Factories

You don't have to stick to carrots in the salad bar, but you should avoid mayonnaise-soaked dishes. Get into the habit of saying, "No cheese" when you order anything they could possibly put cheese on: This simple change could keep thousands of calories a year out of your system. (A single ounce of most hard cheeses has about 100 calories and 10 grams of fat—mostly the saturated kind.) Those unnecessary calories can stay with you as body fat. Theoretically, eating 3,500 calories that you don't burn could add a pound to your body weight. How much anyone actually gains by eating a certain amount of food varies widely depending on many factors. Whatever this elusive number is, it's high, as evidenced by the growing number of obese people.

White chicken meat has fewer calories of fat than darker meat. Cut off the fat-heavy skin of chicken and turkey, and don't eat it.

If you crave a burger, go for the heart-smart meatless variety and dodge a lot of calories, saturated fat, and cholesterol.

79

"Special Request" Meals When Traveling

Your travel agent can easily put your dietary requirements on computer. Then, each time you make a reservation, your reservation automatically assigns you a special meal. These special meals are often outstanding, since they are not made in normal mass production in advance but are specially made each day for those passengers who request them.

On most airlines, you can order the following special meals: Baby, Bland (Low Sodium), Child, Cold Seafood, Diabetic, Fruit Only, Hindu, Kosher, Low-Fat, Moslem, Toddler, Vegetarian (Lacto), and Vegetarian (Pure). (Please note: The children's meals are not necessarily healthy.)

On a recent trip from Tampa to San Francisco, my travel agent ordered "low-fat" meals for me. Here's the comparison of what I ate to the regular meal most other passengers received:

Tampa ───────► Dallas

Normal meal:
- Ham and cheese on a sub roll with mayo
- Bag of Fritos

Nutrition information:
432 calories
24.6 g protein
34 g carbohydrates
22.4 g of fat, of which
5.88 g were saturated

Calories from fat:
47 percent

My low-fat meal:
- Turkey on whole-wheat bread with lettuce
- Low-fat tortilla chips
- Apple

Nutrition information:
338 calories
14.9 g protein
58.3 g carbohydrates
6.67 g of fat, of which
1.34 g were saturated

Calories from fat:
18 percent

Dallas ───────► San Francisco

Normal meal:
- Meat and cheese tortellini in cream sauce
- Salad with Thousand Island dressing
  - Large macadamia nut chocolate chip cookie

My low-fat meal:
- Salad with low-cal ranch dressing
- Chicken breast (3 oz. without skin), with light tomato sauce
- Wild rice and steamed vege-

tables (corn, green beans, broccoli, and cauliflower)
• Pita bread
• Fresh fruit (1/2 apple, 1/3 orange, 2 prunes, and lettuce garnish)

Nutrition information:
580 calories
1,278 mg of sodium,
(53 percent of RDA)
40.8 g protein
97.1 g carbohydrates
5.26 g fat, of which
1.17 g were saturated

Calories from fat:
8 percent

Nutrition information:
1,192 calories
1,577 mg of sodium,
(66 percent of RDA)
37.9 g protein
125 g carbohydrates
61.4 g fat, of which
15.2 were saturated

Calories from fat:
46 percent

Conclusion: Now, the airlines never seem to tire of handing out the little, fat-laden packages of salty peanuts. Without considering the peanuts on the flight, everybody who hadn't special-ordered their meals got food containing 129 percent of their daily RDA for sodium in just two meals. For anyone who has high blood pressure, this is not a great idea. A large number of forty-something and older people have this condition, although many of them don't know it. By contrast, I hit 73 percent of my sodium RDA. However, if I had been concerned about high blood pressure, I also could have ordered low-fat, low-sodium meals and reduced that percentage.

My food contained less than 3 grams of saturated fat, compared to the more than 20 grams most passengers ate. They put away over 1,600 calories (not counting the calories in the alcoholic drinks some of them consumed). I consumed fewer than 1,000 calories.

In terms of the overall quality of the eating experience, I believe my low-fat meals were far superior to the regular menu. All it takes to get in on this good deal is a phone call at least 24 hours before you fly.

Controlling Dehydration Aloft

Never drink alcohol on airplanes unless a specific celebration overrides your concern about what happens to your body. Alcohol causes your body to dehydrate even more than it ordinarily does in a plane's dry air.

Drink juices and water. Stay away from coffee or tea (again, unless you absolutely must have them) because they are diuretics. A diuretic causes you to lose more water than you normally do. Preserve your ability to perform at a high level at your destination; replenish your water instead of losing it by drinking the wrong fluids. Losing significant amounts of water impairs your judgment and makes attaining the Ideal Performance State almost impossible.

What about when the flight attendant comes down the aisle and offers you a drink and a snack? A good rule of thumb is to request a nondiuretic fluid such as juice or sparkling water to replenish your system without bogging you down. You can always get the reliable old standby, plain water, if the cart doesn't carry your favorite item. On many flights, the attendant will offer you peanuts or pretzels. You can probably eat 20 times the amount of pretzels without equaling the fat in one small bag of peanuts.

What about the small cookie, often served as a dessert with inflight meals? It's high sugar, high fat. Leave it on the tray unless you feel like giving yourself a special treat.

Eating on the Run

Everyone reading this book, at one time or another—and probably often—has had to hurry up and eat or go without. Whether it's between sales calls, between meetings, or between appointments, there always seems to be a problem with eating, especially at midday.

When you're on the road in your rental car rushing hurriedly from one meeting to the next, there are times you need to eat and eat fast. And although this philosophy of eating fast does not fit into the Anti-Diet regimen, I recognize there are times you absolutely have to live this lifestyle. Since there's no way around it, here's my recommendation on the quick hits:

Most fast-food chains have a grilled chicken sandwich. When ordering it, make sure you get it with no cheese, mayonnaise, or special sauce. Those special sauces are mostly mayonnaise and usually pack well over 20 grams of fat. Mustard is a great low-fat substitute for special sauces. Many chains also have great salads along with low-fat or fat-free dressings.

So skip the burgers, fish sandwiches, and fries. There's no reason to eat poorly—even when you're running like mad. Anyway, you'd probably rather eat something high in fat at other times, perhaps when you're relaxing with family and friends. Also, there are times when you have no control over what's served, but you do when you're eating on the run. It takes no more than a few seconds to make the healthier choices. Eating on the run is no longer an excuse to eat poorly.

There's nothing wrong with eating at fast-food restaurants, unless all you ever eat there is a burger and fries. Most fast-food restaurants have very healthy selections. Burger King has the BK Broiler, McDonald's has the McGrilled Chicken DeLuxe. Hardee's, Wendy's, and Taco Bell have their versions of the same meal. All these fast-food chains also have very good salad selections (but watch out for the dressing). One very important point in ordering from a fast-food restaurant: Their job is to cater to your taste.

I go to fast-food restaurants quite often because I have two children who like to go there. When ordering I always ask the servers to omit the special sauce. However, like everyone else, I like moisture in my sandwich. So, I often ask for mustard and sometimes ketchup on my sandwiches. Lettuce, tomatoes, and pickles also add to the moisture and flavor of any sandwich.

At hotels and some fast-food restaurants, pizza is a very popular item. A cheese pizza with nothing else on it is about 27 percent fat—not bad for a fast-food restaurant. A hamburger is 56 percent fat.

However, you can do something I find quite tasty. I learned about it by chance while dining at a pizza restaurant with a friend who is lactose intolerant and can't eat cheese. My friend ordered a small pizza with no cheese, but with extra tomato sauce, mushrooms, and other vegetables. This astounded me. I asked the manager if it was a common request. He said, "It happens occasionally, but not too often."

I decided to order the same thing. Yes, I know: We grow up with certain tastes; the idea of a pizza with no cheese seems incredulous. I must tell you, though, it was absolutely terrific. As an extra bonus, it ended up being about 5 to 10 percent fat instead of the 27 to 30 percent fat provided by just the cheeses. (Adding meat to the pizza booms up the fat content even more.)

Many fast-food restaurants have a salad bar (and some even have a pasta bar). Just be wary of the dressing and also of how much butter the pasta in the pasta bar contains. If prepared poorly, a very healthy staple can become unhealthy and loaded with fat.

What If You Absolutely, Positively—No Questions Asked, End of Story—Have to Eat Fast?

Either you're traveling all day long or your day is packed with an impossible amount of demands. In any case, you have to eat on the run, and you simply can't get to great, fresh food.

Here's a sample of what you can do to stay tough on an extra tough day. It's far from the best daily diet, but it will get you through pretty well. This is exactly what Ms. J. Langtry ate on a particularly busy day at the start of a sales trip.

Breakfast—at the Airport
Cinnamon raisin bagel (3 oz.) with cherry/strawberry jam (1 Tbs.)
Coffee (2 cups) and orange juice (8 oz.)
Banana

Midmorning Snack
Apple

Lunch—at a Fast-Food Restaurant
Grilled chicken sandwich (skinless roasted chicken breast, bun, 1 Tbs. mustard)
Tossed green salad (2 cups) with low-fat, oil-free dressing (2 Tbs.)
Low-fat frozen yogurt (1 cup)

Mid-Afternoon Snack—at a Convenience Mart
Banana and an apple

Dinner—at Another Fast-Food Restaurant
2 slices of a 15-inch cheese pizza
Tossed green salad (2 cups) with low-cal French dressing (2 Tbs.)

Dessert
Low-fat frozen yogurt (1 cup)

Analysis of J. Langtry's One-Day Fast-Food Diet:
Age: 50. Gender: female. Weight: 140 lbs. Height: 5 ft. 11 in.
Activity: very active.

Nutritional Category:		*% of RDA*
Calories	2,027	82
Protein	98.7 g	64
Carbohydrates	365 g	107
Fat	27 g	49
Saturated Fat	9.58 g	52
Monounsaturated Fat	8.08 g	44
Polyunsaturated Fat	5.87 g	32
Omega 3 Fat	775 g	—
Omega 6 Fat	4.99 g	—
Cholesterol	117 mg	39
Fiber	26.5 g	107
Vitamin A_1	455 RE	182
A-Rentinol	278 RE	—
A-Carotene	1160 RE	—
B_1-Thiamin	2.1 mg	169
B_2-Riboflavin	2.32 mg	156
B_3-Niacin	31 mg	189
Niacin Equiv.	31 mg	189
Vitamin B_6	2.22 mg	139
Vitamin B_{12}	3.57 mg	179
Folic Acid	563 mg	313
Pantothenic Acid	5.09 mg	73
Vitamin C	171 mg	286
Vitamin D	867 mcg	17
Vitamin E	67 mg	83
Calcium	1355 mg	169
Copper	1.55 mg	62

Iron	14.3 mg	95
Magnesium	385 mg	137
Manganese	2.53 mg	72
Phosphorus	1535 mg	192
Potassium	4519 mg	226
Selenium	88.8 mcg	161
Sodium	3159 mg	132
Zinc	10.3 mg	86

Packing Your Brown Bag for Work

Eat light, eat often, and eat a variety of nonfat or low-fat foods. When you're at work, often the best way is to brown bag it so you can control what you eat. Otherwise the route salesperson for the vending machine down the hall has more control over what you snack on than you do. If you depend on him or her, or on the local fast-food restaurant, the odds are you'll consume large amounts of fat and get very little nutrition. If your workday extends from 7 a.m. to 7 p.m. I recommend never leaving home without a brown bag filled with healthy foods. You may feel less conspicuous by putting the brown bag inside an attaché case or workout bag or keeping it stashed in your desk.

A sliced turkey breast sandwich on rye bread with lettuce, tomato, and mustard is an outstanding lunch. Add a couple of pieces of fruit for fueling your Ferrari the right way at midday.

The brown bag should also contain your midmorning snack and your midafternoon snack. In the midmorning you could have fruit: an apple or peach; a bagel or whole-wheat roll; or cereal in a plastic bag. Any of these would be tremendous. Your midafternoon snack could duplicate the midmorning one. These midmorning and midafternoon snacks serve to stabilize your blood sugar, thus keeping you "up" mentally for the next couple of hours.

If you leave with the family on a long trip, take a brown bag with fruit, whole-grain rolls, fat-free pretzels, rice cakes, and so on. It's a great way to teach your children how to eat for health, longevity, and good appearance.

If the brown-bag concept makes you uncomfortable—an understandable reaction given the importance of image—there are alternatives. You could, for example, have an extra attaché case for food only. A nylon zipper bag might be a good choice. Or you could bring in a few days supply of fruit and keep it in a bowl in your office.

Ordering from Room Service

Eating healthy on the road can be tough. To eat healthy when ordering from room service requires more care than ever. I once flew into a city the evening before I was to give the opening address at a national sales meeting for a multibillion-dollar corporation. I was excited about doing this program and was feeling great. By the time I reached my hotel in a rental car, it was about 8:30 p.m., and I decided to check out the only restaurant still open. What a spread they had set up—their weekly Sunday evening prime-rib buffet. Can you imagine? All the prime rib you can eat.

If I wasn't into this whole lifestyle change, I would have been in that buffet line in a heartbeat (and possibly would have moved a step closer to losing out on many millions of heartbeats as a result). However, I wanted healthier food.

Back in my room, one of the "healthy items" on the room service menu was grilled chicken breast on a whole wheat sourdough bun. It sounded great, so I called in my order and asked (as usual) what came with it. The response was incredible: French fries—on the healthy menu! I told the young lady that I did not want French fries and asked if I could have fruit instead.

"I'm sorry, no substitutions are allowed."

"Just give me the sandwich with no French fries."

Obviously new on the job, she said the French fries came with it.

Instead of arguing, I said, "That's fine." However, I had a taste for some calamari. Although I knew it would probably have too much protein to eat late at night, I hadn't eaten much protein all day. I had snacked throughout the day on healthy carbohydrates, so I felt like I could sway a little bit. The appetizer list in the room service menu had fried calamari. I asked my "friendly" room service person if the calamari could be grilled.

"Of course it can be, sir," she replied in her most helpful

tone, "whatever you want."

That made me very happy. I ordered grilled calamari as an appetizer with a "healthy item" grilled chicken breast sandwich with French fries.

By the time my meal arrived it was well after 9 p.m., and I was very hungry. Both plates on my tray were covered. Under one cover I saw my wonderful grilled chicken breast sandwich (no mayonnaise, of course) with the fries I never wanted. Then I removed the second cover and found breaded and deep-fried calamari—a nightmare of fat.

Now I had to think. Do I pass on the calamari, or do I say, "The heck with it," and just eat it? I really wanted the calamari, but I also really wanted to eat healthy. So I rationalized: Calamari is not a porous food. It's tough, almost rubberlike in texture, so it shouldn't absorb much fat from the grease it was cooked in. That's all it took. I ate some of the calamari one by one, but only after peeling all the breading off. It sure tasted good, but my fingers were one big glob of grease when I was through. (That's why I only ate a few.)

How to Beat the Midafternoon Trough

The ten-round fight to avoid being knocked out by the midafternoon trough starts the day before. Round 1 sees you getting in a physical workout to recover from the day's mental and emotional stress. Round 2, you eat dinner early. Round 3, you get a good night's sleep. Round 4, you eat a nutritious breakfast. Round 5 is your midmorning snack. Choose something, preferably an apple or other fruit, to maintain your blood sugar level and keep you from getting so hungry that you'll eat too much at lunch time.

In Round 6 you're at a restaurant, where you help steer your group's conversation toward relaxation and fun and away from heavy, worrisome, stressful subjects. You can't beat good cheer as a digestive and recovery aid at mealtime. If you're mentally tough, you've progressed well beyond the immature concept that reaching good cheer requires alcohol. When the server sounds the gong for Round 7 by asking for drink orders "to start with," opt for something nonalcoholic, even if it's plain water. Round 8 sees you ordering a low-fat meal of about two to three parts complex carbohydrates to two parts protein. In Round 9, you decline having an alcoholic beverage with lunch and concentrate instead on enjoying your food and companions. As Round 10 starts, you're feeling well-recovered, and you skip the high-fat or sugary desserts. For your after-lunch drink, you order mineral water instead of alcohol or, if you tolerate caffeine well, coffee or tea.

If you keep on punching for high afternoon alertness all the way through Round 10, I guarantee your afternoon productivity and performance won't hit the canvas. While the rest of the gang is drowsing through the midafternoon trough, you'll be getting things done, making points, and moving ahead with your career. Your knockout punch is the healthy snack you eat at the office around 3:30 p.m.

Winning Tactics at Pit Stops

Even though chocolate chip cookies and small bags of potato chips are tempting, choose pretzels or fruit instead. This is your life. Today counts! In fact, today is all we ever have. You can't do anything about what you ate yesterday, and tomorrow isn't here yet. Focus on what you eat today, and how slim you look tomorrow will take care of itself.

For your second, fourth, and sixth meals of the day (breakfast is first, lunch third, and dinner fifth) here's a list of healthy snacks:

Apples	Nuts
Bagels	Oranges
Bananas	Pears
Berries	Plums
Broccoli	Popcorn (air-popped)
Carrots	Pretzels
Cauliflower	Radishes
Celery	Raisins
Cherries	Skim Milk
Fig Newtons	Soups
Fruit Juices	Cherry Tomatoes
Grapes	Yogurt (low-fat frozen)
Melon	

The Business Dinner

Be careful when eating out. Many restaurants have a "healthy menu," but the items they list may not be the best foods for you. Some healthy items on menus still are extremely high in fat. The best Anti-Dieting thing to do at any restaurant also impresses the client: Never open the menu. Simply decide what you would like to eat beforehand and ask them to fix it. You might decide on grilled chicken breast on a rice pilaf, grilled chicken with pasta, or sliced turkey with marinara sauce on whole-wheat bread with lettuce, tomato, and mustard.

If you feel compelled to eat red meat, ask the server if the restaurant has veal because it's lower in fat than mature beef. If your client orders dessert and you feel compelled to have dessert, ask for fresh berries or fresh fruit. If unavailable, ask for a small piece of angel food cake or a small dish of sherbet.

When your client orders a Caesar salad, you can simply order a lettuce and tomato salad with your dressing on the side. Then minimize the fat from the salad dressing by dipping your fork vertically in the salad dressing (no scooping allowed). This leaves enough dressing on the prongs of the fork to get the taste of the dressing without the incredibly high caloric (and usually fat) content of the dressing.

Simply refuse to feel pressure from clients to order a lot of alcohol and red meat. If you want to join them in a drink, order a glass of wine and sip on it the entire evening.

When You Have No Choice

In the winter of 1982, I conducted a tennis clinic at a beautiful indoor club near Boston. In my address to 40 junior athletes and their parents, I bestowed my then-current thinking about proper nutrition.

I denounced saturated fat as being almost an evil (which in some ways I still feel it is), but I failed to regard human behavior modification in my presentation. I told the attendees to get off red meat, since it was not what their bodies could utilize effectively. One man there was of special note: Russ Adams, an internationally renowned tennis photographer.

It was the year of my awakening to an important fact: In some circumstances, it's virtually impossible to go totally cold turkey on some foods. At the U.S. Open tennis tournament later that year, I arrived at the site at 9 a.m. to watch some of my players practice for their 11 a.m. matches. I had eaten a good breakfast at 7:30, but I hadn't prepared at all for the day ahead. From 11:00 a.m. to about 2 p.m. I watched a men's match, and then I had another player competing in just a few minutes.

I was famished and needed to eat something. The concession stand offered no salads, no lean meats, and no vegetables. Here I was—a guy who espouses the virtues of healthy eating to the tennis community. At the U.S. Open Food Court back then, the only foods were burgers, dogs, and fries. What should I do? I now laugh at the dilemma I was faced with.

I needed to eat—anything! So, I casually went up to the food counter and ordered a hamburger—those burgers were huge! I walked quickly away from the food court to find a quiet and suitably private place to eat my sinister hamburger. Under a stairwell at the U.S. Open I found a crate to sit on and got ready to "scarf" down my sandwich. So here I was—hiding at the world's biggest tennis tournament with 30,000 people all around me—eating a burger.

I had only been there a few seconds when around the corner of the stairwell, within five feet of me, came Russ Adams. You have no idea how embarrassed I felt when Russ said in his most jovial voice, "Wow, this could be a fun photo to have!" He teasingly raised his camera and said, "Hey, there's nothing wrong with a little red meat now and then." His sagacious remark reached me at the right moment in my career. He was right!

Russ and I laugh about it to this day. There truly is nothing wrong with having a little red meat occasionally. The key point is *don't hide to eat or be a closet junkie with your food.* When you want something, eat it. However, if it's not very good for you, eat it only in moderation.

Chapter 6

CUTTING OUT THE FAT

*"Americans have the highest amount of fat intake
anywhere in the world."*
—Tom Brokaw, NBC Nightly News,
Jan. 24, 1996

While having a leisurely weekend breakfast recently, a well-dressed, heavy-set man in his thirties at the next table caught my attention when he made a phone call. Then his breakfast arrived. I watched in amazement as the server placed enough food for three people in front of him.

He had ordered a full stack of pancakes, ham and eggs, hash browns, toast, and coffee, to which he added cream and sugar. He finished before I did. When he got up and lumbered off, I saw that he had left nothing on his plates but the melon slice that had come with his food. Clearly, if it wasn't fat-heavy, he wouldn't eat it.

Without even speaking to the man, or knowing anything of his circumstances other than what I could see, it was obvious that he was racing toward a health disaster, probably a heart attack before he was 45.

By definition, a business executive is someone who takes charge, prioritizes, gets things done, and exerts authority. So it's surprising to see how few executives include their personal health in the projects they give high priority to—until they get a wake-up call in the form of a personal medical emergency.

Strange, isn't it? By any logical standard, work pressure has to rank several orders of magnitude below the importance of simply staying alive. Make no mistake about it: The most important element in determining your future health and longevity consists of how well you manage your personal health—*you*, not your spouse, not your doctor. You can't evade your responsibility for keeping yourself alive. As members of the animal kingdom, eating wisely and being active are our best hopes for surviving and thriving.

If your blood cholesterol is out of control, little plaques of the stuff accumulate along the walls of your arteries with the inevitability of taxes and compound interest. For this reason, you can't start too early to slow or reverse the process. Yes, with adequate exercise—and by eating nutritiously and avoiding much of the popular high-fat, high-cholesterol foods—you can stop or reverse your slide toward cardiovascular disease. Research bears this out.

Cholesterol Is an Animal Product

Dietary cholesterol is very different from blood serum cholesterol, and some research shows that dietary cholesterol is not something to concern yourself with. However, this research is not yet definitive, so I recommend that you keep control of your dietary cholesterol intake.

What you want to achieve is a low consumption of dietary cholesterol each day. If you were a pure vegetarian—no milk, no eggs, no meat or animal products—you would not get any cholesterol in your diet. Cholesterol is only found in animal products.

Cholesterol is essential to health, but your body makes all it needs. This means that when you eat more of it, you risk running into a dangerous oversupply. You should eat no more than 300 milligrams of cholesterol a day.

Low-density lipoproteins (LDLs) are the bad cholesterol responsible for the blood-flow-reducing buildup along arterial walls. High-density lipoproteins (HDLs) are the good cholesterol.

Triglycerides are fats in the blood.

Saturated fats, such as those found in meats, solidify at room temperature. Saturated fats aren't good at all. They cause a significant increase in LDL and triglycerides.

Monounsaturated fats, found in olive oil, are excellent. Using olive oil for cooking is a tremendous health builder.

Monounsaturated fats cause a significant increase in HDL and a moderate decrease in LDL and triglycerides.

Omega-3 fats, found in seafood, reduce the risk of blood clots that could trigger a heart attack by blocking a coronary artery. They're effective, and you can easily obtain all the benefit that omega-3 fats provide from food. You shouldn't need a supplement. Taking omega-3 pills is a waste of money, a fact research has established.

Hydrogenated oils are treated vegetable oils that your body responds to exactly the same as saturated fat. Don't be fooled by the words "vegetable" or "soybean" and so on. If *hydrogenated* or *partially hydrogenated* precedes the item, the word "hydrogenated" means it's bad.

How Frying Can Clog Your Arteries

Have you ever fried a steak, hamburger, pork, or lamb in a pan? As soon as the meat was fried, you probably served it and let the pan sit to cool. When you came back, what did the substance in the cooled pan look like?

It was white and solid, wasn't it? That's because it's saturated fat. Some fast-food restaurants still get the fat they fry French fries in from their frying pans, which accounts for the high-fat content of their fries. They do it because the saturated fat is a cost-free waste product. Instead of spending money to get rid of it, they save money by using it for frying French fries.

Gradually, some of the better-run outlets switched to tropical oils, which were no better from the saturated fat standpoint. Then many people learned how dangerous it could be to eat saturated fat-fried potatoes, and sales dropped. The big hamburger markets quickly caved in to public opinion. Now you can be reasonably sure that French fries from a chain outlet have been fried in vegetable oil (hopefully not the hydrogenated kind) rather than in saturated fat from animals or cheap tropical oils.

Years ago, many people poured the residue of saturated fat from their frying pans into a can for later use in frying vegetables, but most home cooks know better today. Now they use an unsaturated vegetable oil such as olive oil, corn oil, safflower oil, or canola oil.

You're enlightened about saturated fat, so you want to get rid of the solid greasy white stuff in your pan. But if you heat it up again to make it liquid and pour it down the drain, you might clog the drain. To unclog it, you might need Drano or some other powerful chemical cleaner—or call the plumber.

Likewise, if you eat a lot of meat that is high in saturated fat, you may have to unclog your drains (your coronary arteries) by calling a "plumber" (a thoracic surgeon) to perform open-heart surgery to either bypass the blocked arteries or to scrape them out at a staggering cost—along with the chilling risk of damaging the arteries. But at least you'll live a little longer: In the best hospitals, 98 out of 100 people undergoing bypass operations survive at least long enough to leave the hospital.

What Ham, Eggs, and Steak Do to Your Arteries

Now, there's nothing wrong with steak or red meat in small amounts. But consider this all-too-common diet for one day. *Breakfast*: ham and eggs (either one alone is high in fat and cholesterol). *Lunch*: cheeseburger with fries and a soft drink. (Groan). *Dinner*: T-bone steak and shrimp combination with butter dip, a baked potato drowned in butter and sour cream, and cheesecake for dessert. (Unspeakable.)

Here's how this fatty diet compares to the Recommended Daily Allowances for a healthy 2,000 calorie diet:

Item	Healthy Diet	Fatty Diet
Calories	2,000	2,422
Cholesterol	200 mg	875 mg
Total Fat	44 g	140 g
Saturated Fat	5 g	61 g
Carbohydrates	250 g	183 g
Protein	150 g	110 g

Probably few corporate executives would show the total ignorance of health considerations it would take to eat three fat-loaded meals in one day. However, many regularly consume two meals a day just as lethal as those given above and think nothing of it. This diet, repeated month after month, is risky to say the least. It is especially risky for business people who are typically mentally overtrained and physically undertrained. The odds of surviving such a high-fat diet until retirement are not good.

Does Cholesterol Deserve Its Bad Rap?

Within limits, blood cholesterol level can be a good predictor of heart attack risk. People who eat the Mediterranean diet can have a rate of coronary heart disease half what their cholesterol level predicted. But few Americans move to Crete, adopt the traditional Mediterranean diet, or take up the backbreaking labor involved in unmechanized methods of farming. Unless you do that, cholesterol deserves the bad rap it gets in this country.

How can you stay here, continue your present lifestyle with only minor changes, and still dodge the dangers of cholesterol? Here's how to do it:

1. Eat no more than 4 ounces of red meat no more than twice a week.
2. Take butter and mayonnaise out of your diet.
3. Get 40 to 50 percent of your calories from fruits, vegetables, and whole grains.
4. Get most of your protein from fish and poultry.
5. Minimize the saturated fat in your diet. Note that it's *saturated* fat you want to minimize; not *monounsaturated* fat, which your body utilizes well. Monounsaturated fat should comprise about 10 percent of your total nutritional intake.

More Cholesterol Where You Least Expect It: Lean Meat

The cholesterol is in the meat, not just in the visible fat that marbles the choicest cuts. This means that the cholesterol is still there, no matter how lean the cut. Lean meat is better for you, but it's better because it has fewer grams of fat, not less cholesterol.

Amazingly, in this day of widespread concern over health costs, the government still reserves the *Choice* designation for meat that's heavily marbled with fat and has the greatest potential for clogging arteries. Those responsible for the continuation of that policy apparently are far removed from the government's budget dilemmas over the soaring costs of health care.

Take the High-Fat Curse Off Ground Meat

At the University of Minnesota, researchers have developed an easy method to take the curse of excessive fat off the popular ground meat. Here's how you do it: Brown the ground meat in a non-stick pan and then drain off the fat. Place the meat in a mesh strainer, pour hot water over it, and allow it to drain. This process reduces the fat content of ordinary ground beef from nearly 30 percent of total weight to less than 10 percent.

However, draining away most of the fat also washes away some of the flavor. You can train yourself to prefer low-fat ground meat, especially when you consider that eating healthy prevents fat from taking up permanent residence along the walls of your coronary arteries. Since meat doesn't stay together as well without fat to bind it (it works the same way in the pan as it does in your heart) it's best in tacos, casseroles, chili, and spaghetti sauce.

Fighting Fat for Your Family and Your Life

Monounsaturated fats, especially olive oil, are excellent nutritionally, being a great source of the fat your body needs. Monounsaturated fats cause a significant increase in HDL (good cholesterol) and a moderate decrease in LDL (bad cholesterol) and triglycerides.

Eating one or two servings of any fish weekly is associated with lower risk of heart disease, certainly a matter that should concern every Corporate Athlete. Research indicates that the higher the fat content of the fish, the greater the cardiovascular benefit. Fish with moderate to high fat content include freshwater bass, bluefish, carp, catfish, halibut, herring, mackerel, mullet, ocean perch, orange roughy, pompano, rainbow trout, salmon, sardines, shad, and smelt.

Trim and discard any visible fat and the liver of the fish, and don't eat the skin because pollutants or contaminants tend to be concentrated in those areas. The omega-3 fats that provide the greatest cardiovascular benefits are found throughout the flesh of cooked seafood and are retained well in most canned fish.

Know What's in the Food You Eat

Unless you know what's in the food you eat, you risk putting sludge in your Ferrari's tank. If you've done that all your life, it's important to start improving your fueling methods right away.

One egg is 65 percent fat and 1 percent carbohydrate. A steak with all the fat trimmed is still 62 percent fat and 0 carbohydrate. But a salad with 2 cups of lettuce, 2 tablespoons of chopped tomatoes, 2 tablespoons of grated carrots, and no dressing is 10 percent fat and only 43 calories.

Now let's add 2 tablespoons of the average low-calorie dressing. The bad news is this innocent little salad then shoots up sharply in fat and calories. You almost quadruple the fat and double the calories with low-fat salad dressing.

Many people claim they can't lose weight no matter how they eat. Aside from exercising far less than they think they do, these people generally defeat their weight-loss efforts with easily overlooked habits, such as ignoring the fat and calorie content of salad dressings, loading their baked potatoes with fat-heavy butter, sour cream, or bacon bits, and disregarding the empty calories of soft and hard drinks.

Tasty salad dressings with zero fat are in the supermarkets now, and alternatives are available for the other overlooked sources of fat just mentioned. Everyone who is serious about losing weight should make healthy changes in all these areas.

There is very little nutrition in dressing—I've searched because I like dressing! I always order dressing on the side, or if I can't get it that way, I push the dressing to the side of the plate. I dab my fork in it and leave most of the dressing on the plate, but I still get enough for taste. I encourage you to try it.

Nutrition Labeling

Now let's talk about one of the best things for consumers to come out of government in a long time: nutrition labeling. This initiative was spearheaded by Phil Sokolof of Omaha, the man who, a few years ago, took on McDonald's and other fast-food chains with full-page ads saying they were poisoning America. With that fight won, Phil moved on to food labeling.

The new nutrition labeling act turns a pitiless spotlight on how bad some foods are for you. Not surprisingly, the food industry is doing its best to minimize the damage and still stay within the law. Their main tool of deception is "serving size." By cutting serving sizes in half, they cut the Percent Daily Value in half—the number they believe most label checkers look at. Candy bars are a good example. Some of them claim that each bar contains two or more servings, even though they know most people eat the whole bar at one time. A small, 8-ounce can of pork and beans claims two servings, so they can legally assert that one serving supplies only 490 milligrams of sodium, which is 21 percent of your RDA. But if you put away the whole can, you consume 42 percent of your daily allotment of salt.

The One-Minute Nutrition Label Analyzer

A nutrition label says a hot dog is 92 percent fat-free, but by reading its label we calculate that it's 87 percent fat! Two-percent milk contains 27 percent fat!

This is all marketing. These deceiving numbers are calculated by the volume of water taken off, for example, when a hot dog is measured by water volume. The water obviously has fat, but the solid that makes the hot dog when it's in its casing is still very high in fat—87 percent!

The key element is serving size. The Percent Daily Value on the label shows what you get by eating one serving of the food in question, but if you ordinarily eat two or three servings of the food at a time, double or triple the Percent Daily Value.

If a milk label says it has 11 grams of carbohydrates and 8 grams each of fat and protein, that looks good on the surface. However, there are 9 calories in each gram of fat, but only 4 calories in each gram of protein or carbohydrate. This means you can eat twice as much protein and carbohydrate as fat without taking in more calories.

Now let's look at that glass of milk. Eleven grams of carbohydrates, multiplied by four, is 44 calories; the protein is another 32 calories. However, the fat's eight grams, multiplied by nine calories per gram, is a whopping 72 calories. Dividing fat calories by total calories (148) gives the percentage of fat. In this case, we see that 49 percent of the calories in whole, pasteurized milk comes from fat, and it is mostly saturated—the worst kind. Whole milk is almost half saturated fat! By comparison, skim milk has less than half a gram of fat per cup, almost twice as much calcium, and only 1/7th as much cholesterol as whole milk. Skim milk is a tremendous food; it's not calorically dense, but it's loaded with good nutrients.

You should choose foods that have low or zero percentages of saturated fat.

Filter Your Coffee to Avoid Raising Your Cholesterol

Recent research conducted in Sweden and Finland has established a strange fact: Drinking boiled, unfiltered coffee can raise your blood cholesterol. This danger seems to be averted by drip-filtered coffee. This process may filter out a still unidentified cholesterol-boosting substance.

Perhaps you're hung up on preparing coffee with a filterless method such as boiling, steeping, or percolating. If so, the best available knowledge powerfully urges the simple operation of passing the brew through a filter to eliminate this risk.

Conquering the Caffeine Curse

Many people rely on coffee to get them going in the morning or to pick them up during the workday. Probably most of them realize they are trying to make a drug achieve what only adequate sleep can accomplish. They probably also know that substituting caffeine for sleep month after month will make them look older fast. They know all this, yet even in this youth-oriented culture of ours, they continue a practice that speeds the aging process while helping to prevent them from reaching their greatest potential.

Where do you start to break an excessive reliance on the caffeine jolt? If you're one of those night owls who believes that you function best on considerably less than eight hours of sleep combined with a caffeine jump start, or if you feel that it's stylish or cute to fumble until midmorning, the first step is to rid yourself of those delusions. Success at this depends on reorganizing your life to get adequate sleep.

If you can't live without the late-night shows, program

your VCR and watch them a day late at dinnertime. Can't fall asleep early? Join a health club and recover from the mental stresses of the day through exercise. The healthy, pleasant feeling of fatigue you'll get with the proper amount of exercise will make it much easier to fall asleep promptly.

Do whatever it takes, but get enough sleep so you wake up in the morning feeling rested and eager for the day. With adequate exercise and rest, your craving for caffeine will diminish or even vanish.

Head Off Headaches with Wise Food Choices, Not Pills

Headaches—the real ones, not just the metaphorical ones so often bandied about—are common in the corporate world. "Too much stress," people commonly say. Well, there may be other reasons, like what you eat and drink, how much you eat and drink, and when you eat and drink.

The main culprits, according to the National Headache Foundation, are chocolate in any form, beer, red wine, aged cheeses, avocados, and overripe bananas. All of them contain tyramine, an amino acid that runs wild in your head, causing some brain blood vessels to dilate and others to constrict, which brings on the headache.

So, before you reach for the latest pill touted on TV, or for your long-time favorite headache remedy, consider your food and drink intake. Does it make any sense to eat or drink something that disturbs your brain flow so much you have to take a pill to counteract it?

A few foods can even cause headaches. If you have frequent headaches and have already considered the common culprits, consider avoiding foods containing the additives Yellow Dye Number 5 or the notorious Monosodium Glutamate (MSG). An allergy to MSG can be serious, even life-threatening. Many people who don't have a full-blown allergy to MSG just get a bad headache from the stuff, often found in Chinese food.

If you have been in the habit of consuming a lot of caffeine, cutting it out suddenly can cause headaches. If you suspect caffeine, taper off slowly. Replace coffee and tea with decaffeinated drinks, and fruit juices for soft drinks. Don't overlook cutting back on the caffeine in chocolate.

Can a Drink Now and Then Help—or Is This Hogwash?

Good news with beer—there's no fat. The bad news is that beer has 62 percent wasted (nutritionless) calories. So, out of all the alcoholic drinks, beer is the healthiest nutritionally because it's 36 percent carbohydrates. One beer or one glass of wine every day is no problem, according to the scientific literature, but more tends to create stress.

Red wine, fat-free and with ten percent carbohydrates, was briefly touted as a miracle weapon against heart disease. This happened after researchers noted that French people, who typically drink red wine with their meals, have a remarkably lower heart disease rate than Americans in spite of eating a diet even heavier in saturated fats. Subsequent studies revealed that the French diet has only recently moved into the high saturated fat range, meaning millions of today's French adults grew up eating a far healthier diet than they do today. As a result, their heart disease rates are creeping up as their levels of artery-clogging begin to match ours. In other words, it wasn't the wine but the diet.

Some research suggests that one or two drinks a day might not harm health, but more stresses the liver and opens the door to a host of other problems.

So, on the basis of present-day research, we can say it might not be hogwash to assert that one drink a day provides health benefits. However, compelling evidence exists to prove this contention: Consistently drinking more than three ounces of alcohol a day decreases performance and longevity.

Here is a summary of the nutritionless calories in some popular alcoholic drinks—the sips that stay on your hips:

Beverage	Serving Size (oz.)	Calories
80-proof hard liquor	1	100-110
Beer	12	150
Bloody Mary	2	116
Daquiri	2	111
Gin and Tonic	7.5	171
Manhattan	2	128

Martini	2.5	156
Pina Colada	4.5	262
Screwdriver	7	174
Sherry	3	126
Stout on tap	12	200
Tequila Sunrise	5.5	189
Tom Collins	7.5	121
Wine	5	105

Sixty-five percent of the executives surveyed in my seminars say they drink more than three ounces of alcohol a day. This doesn't bode well against the prevailing research. Consuming no more than two ounces of alcohol daily may actually help your general health, according to several research studies, but there are compelling data in the same research that shows you're taking risks by drinking close to the limit—or habitually exceeding it. Such research has revealed a narrow dividing line between benefit and damage. As soon as you go beyond two ounces: boom—you're beyond what your body can handle without damage. That's how drastic the division is and how quickly the line between helpfulness and overstress from alcohol gets passed.

"Blood pressure is exquisitely sensitive to alcohol," says Paul Whelton of Johns Hopkins University. "The evidence is consistent and powerful."

William Haskell of Stanford University maintains you don't have to abstain from alcohol to avoid high blood pressure. "There's no good evidence one or two drinks a day have much effect on blood pressure," Haskell says. "Only those who drink more than two alcoholic beverages a day will substantially raise their risk of high blood pressure."

A small amount of alcohol, even on a daily basis, has been shown by many health organizations to be okay, even beneficial. Some researchers have found that one or two drinks a day can raise HDL levels by up to 20 percent. However, losing excess weight and engaging in physical activity can also raise HDL levels by up to 20 percent. Weight loss and exercise also provide other benefits that alcohol can't match, such as reducing the risk of diabetes, causing the heart to work more efficiently, and decreasing blood pressure. Moderation is the key to preventing alcohol from hammering our livers, interfering with our mental functions, and doing weird things to our lives. For many people who may have a genetic predilection toward alcoholism, even a sip is too much because they can't stop there.

According to many authorities, moderate drinking means no more than two ounces a day for men of average size and only one ounce for women of average size. Obviously, a 105-pound woman has less body mass to dilute two ounces of alcohol than a 160-pound man. For anyone taking prescription drugs, however, drinking any alcohol at all may be very dangerous.

Why Couch Potatoes Die Young

The worst-case couch potatoes start dying in their 30s, but the large-scale stampede to the graveyard starts when they are in their 40s. By that time many of them have been underexercising and overeating for 20 years or more. Now that children become couch potatoes at ever younger ages, death rates among them will also begin to peak in even younger adult years.

The causes of couch-potato death are variously given: heart attack and other cardiovascular diseases, such as coronary thrombosis, and a wide variety of cancers. Since couch potatoes tend to prefer fat-saturated, salty foods and avoid fruits and vegetables, they are at high risk for colon or rectal cancers.

Lung and throat cancers are frequently represented because many couch potatoes speed their dash to the grave by adding tobacco to their other self-inflicted wounds. However, the true cause of death—not cancer, heart attack, or stroke—never appears on their death certificates since the true killer is not a recognized disease. It can be summed up in one word: *lifestyle*. But that's a misnomer for couch potatoes because they don't have a lifestyle, they live a *death style*.

What a tragedy! Many of them live just long enough to acquire a spouse and children, so the loss is not to themselves alone—the greater pain and loss is suffered by the loved ones who are left behind to fend for themselves.

Chapter 7

TRAINING YOUR BODY TO BE ENERGETIC, AND ENJOY DOING IT

"Vigorous exercise is as important as not being overweight and not smoking in lengthening life."
—I-Min Lee

Most people have trouble maintaining an exercise program. All but the most devout health nuts have problems getting motivated and started on some days.

This chapter is for the people who must get started, and stay motivated, to perform better on the job and in their private life every day. The good news is that you can train your body to be slim and energetic, and you can love doing it, too. The bad news is that you have to want it for yourself, for your own reasons, and you must have a sharp hunger for it. Otherwise, you'll fight it all the way, and nothing will change much. It can't be someone else's idea—someone else nagging you to do it. *You* have to want to change.

Why Would You Want to Change?

If you become more energetic, you'll enjoy your work more, and you'll have enough stamina left at the end of the day to enjoy your family and free time more. Your self-esteem will expand, your confidence will grow, and your performance will soar. You will feel like you're in control of your life because you'll be far more in control than you possibly could be while hauling pounds of excess body fat every step you take. We've seen it happen with thousands of businesspeople who became mentally tough enough to improve their lean body mass-to-fat ratio, thereby boosting their stamina. With entire companies going on this program, the total amount of weight shifted from body fat to lean muscle mass literally runs into the tons. It adds up to an enormous increase in productive capacity, fitness, and health.

My recommendation is to take on energizing your mind and body as a business project and set it up like any other important project. It's difficult to imagine a more important personal project than increasing your physical and mental energy. Gaining more stamina will make all your other goals much easier to achieve.

It's Never Too Late

If you're overweight and over 40, don't lull yourself to sleep (the long, final sleep) by thinking, "It won't do any good to change now; it's too late for me."

The body will adapt physically and mentally at any age. As long as you're still breathing, it's not too late to make significant progress at boosting your stamina and extending your life. This has been proven by studies conducted among people in their 90s. One group exercised with weights; the control group did nothing new. After a year, the exercisers had increased their mobility, strength, and mental alertness significantly compared to the control group—at 90 years old! So don't take the "It's too late for me" copout—unless you're over 130. "It ain't over 'til it's over."

Resistance to Change

Let's take a closer look at the key to the problem: your innate resistance to change. We must consider its two parts: your mind's attitude, and your body's set point.

Your attitude can be deceptive. Most of us tend to think we can simply decide to change how we do something, and bang—it's done. Often it's not easy because our decisions can be overwhelmed by other pressures and demands.

Study your lifestyle carefully before trying to raise your stamina. Allow for some backsliding. Anticipate having to fight off temptations to quit. Expect to readjust until you hit a workable schedule and formula. Count on it; you'll hit plateaus where progress seems to stall. Now you must tune in intently to your body's signals. The vital thing is to do a little more each week until your body tells you to ease up.

If you haven't been exercising or if you are older than 30, get your doctor's approval first. Then start with three workouts a week, each session lasting between 30 and 45 minutes. Don't fall into the trap of thinking one long workout a week is as good as three shorter ones spaced throughout the week. The difference is recovery. One workout a week is an open invitation to problems ranging from aches and pains to heart attacks; three milder workouts a week put you on the road to greater energy, stamina, and longevity.

Your body's set point can be far more stubborn than your attitude, but you can change it. Your body's set point is the point at which the body resists losing weight. It does this by slowing its metabolic rate to use food more efficiently. This automatic survival technique helps people survive in the under-fed third world; however, it's counterproductive for nearly everyone in the industrialized world, where it causes overfed people to store more fat than they will ever need.

Exercising Safely at Any Age

People hear from every side about getting a checkup before embarking on an exercise program. However, if they follow the life-threatening lifestyle of not exercising at all, no physical checkup is necessary.

Getting a checkup is excellent advice for any sedentary person thinking about exercising. This is especially important for anyone over 45 who is at high risk because of obesity, smoking, diabetes, high blood cholesterol, hypertension, severe stress, or a family history of medical problems. So, if you decide to protect your health with exercise, by all means get all the medical help you can to prolong your life.

Warm Up to Exercise

Warm up right. The body—even a well-conditioned one—is like a big container of lard. The tissues are not soft and pliable; they're tight and rigid. Heating your body does the same thing to your tissues as heating a pan of lard. It softens and makes the tissues more flexible. Adequate warm-up is vital for everyone before exercise, but especially so for the poorly conditioned or for those who are older. By getting your body ready for the more strenuous exercise to come, the warm-up greatly reduces the chances of injury.

Adequate warm-ups have two parts:

1. ***Break a sweat.*** Walk briskly, cycle, or run in place or on a treadmill until you start sweating.

2. ***Stretch.*** Run through your stretch routine so your body will be as flexible as possible for your heavy exercise session.

Variety is the spice of life. Walk or run on the level, hike in the hills, ride a bicycle, row, use a step machine, lift weights, swim, play tennis or racquetball, ski on snow or water—the possibilities are endless.

Develop the right mental attitude. Don't try to whip yourself into terrific shape overnight. Avoid overtraining because it leads to injuries. However, as you find your body growing stronger, make sure you get out of your comfort zone a little, and then get recovery.

Go slow; getting fit is like a marathon, not a sprint. It took a lot of time to get to your current fitness level. So, if you're out of shape, take your time to get back in shape. Moving deliberately toward fitness is the quickest way to get there.

Build Muscle to Burn Fat Faster

Pound for pound, muscle burns fat faster than fat burns fat. According to William Kraemer of Pennsylvania State University, "For every pound of muscle you gain, you will burn an extra 30 to 50 calories per day." When you exercise, your muscles work while your body fat just goes along for the ride.

Doesn't some fat get burned when I exercise?

Yes, but only a tiny amount. Mainly you burn carbohydrates. Your next meal replaces those carbohydrates, and most likely, the fat you just burned, too. Exercise isn't a major factor in weight loss, but it's the main factor in preventing weight gain or regain.

What? I thought exercise was essential to weight loss.

It is, in a roundabout way and over the long haul. Muscle

burns more fat 24 hours a day, and you burn most of your calories and fat when you're not exercising. The more muscle you have, the more fat you burn.

The exercise machines and charts reporting how many calories are burned per hour with a particular exercise grossly underestimate the effect of physical training. The higher rate of calorie burning continues long after the exercise stops. Active bodies have a higher metabolic rate than sedentary bodies; they not only burn more fat by expending more energy, they burn it faster, and keep on burning it faster, even during sleep.

I'm not seriously overweight; I just have this flat tire around my middle. What's the best way to get rid of it?

With a two-pronged attack: One, reduce your fat intake by eating fewer and better calories. Two, exercise aerobically and use strength training to build your health, increase your productivity, and burn more fat. Since you burn most of your calories at rest (about 60-70 percent), you must develop muscle to help your program.

A good weight-training routine stresses all the major muscle groups. Working out at least twice a week can significantly improve your body's tone and cause it to burn more calories.

Can't I just eat less fat?

Sure you can, and you'll lose a little—until your body adjusts to your lower fat intake by slowing your metabolism. People who only diet and avoid exercising just lose weight for a while. After losing a few pounds, they stop losing weight; they may even slowly regain every pound they've lost.

I want quick results. I plan to cut my fat intake to zero.

Don't do it. Eat about 20 percent fat because your body must have some fat for many essential purposes. Since the membranes between your cells and most of the cells in your brain and nervous system are composed of fat, one of the body's needs is to replenish those areas. A strict no-fat diet not only endangers your health, it's also incredibly difficult to maintain. You'll get quicker results by eating right and exercising more.

With every decade of life after age 30, you lose 10 percent of your muscle mass and a similar percent of brain capacity. This is true of the body only if you do not engage in regular strength training, and of the brain only if you do not engage in mental effort and exercises to enhance your intellectual energy.

The one percent a year loss of muscle mass means that by the time you're 40 you will have lost 10 percent of your muscle mass. If you don't strength train, by the time you're 50 you will have lost another 10 percent. It keeps going, which is why some older people are so frail, although it's not unusual for long-term weight lifters to be stronger at 75 than nonexercising men half their age.

Even moderate amounts of strength training over relatively short periods of time have been shown to be amazingly beneficial. Sixty-year-old people were studied by the University of Colorado. After strength training for one year, the 60-year-olds had increased their muscle mass. They also had more muscle-building hormones than 20-year-olds who were sedentary.

The Link Between Physical and Mental Toughness

Physical toughening makes it easier to access the Ideal Performance State (IPS) and to discover your ultimate potential. The mind and body are one. Exercising the right way will train your body's physiological response to mental and emotional stress. This is why any athlete who hopes for mental toughening must begin physical toughening as well.

When confronted by a formidable task or stressful situation, you have felt challenged rather than threatened, haven't you? You've loved the fight. It may have happened in sports, business, or in life when you were opposed by someone or something. Instead of finding the opposition threatening, you found it challenging. Responding to a challenge with the fight response releases catecholamine hormones and activates IPS. Catecholamines create the "fight response" in your system.

In the corporate world, and very likely in our families, too, fear often exists. Children may fear someone at school or be afraid to try out for a sport, the band, or a chorus. Some tasks at work create the fear response because we may not feel we can live up to expectations. When you have the fear response to a challenge, massive amounts of cortisol flow into your bloodstream. This hormone is responsible for the "fight or flight," or fear response. For this reason we view excessive amounts of cortisol as negative.

The Hormone Factor

To see what physical toughening will do for you in this area, let's examine the hormonal response to exercise:

Exercise increases catecholamine production capacity, thus providing the material for catecholamine spikes. Over time, exercise increases the catecholamine response so you spike faster. Exercise also lowers your resting level of catecholamines, preparing the way for quicker spikes, and it speeds catecholamine recovery to low resting levels, so future challenges are met sooner and more effectively by new catecholamine spikes.

Exercise lowers resting levels and provides higher capacity, faster spikes, and quicker recoveries. Aren't these results the way you want to respond to stress? When hit in the face emotionally, you'll respond with a quick spike of catecholamines. This causes you to feel like saying, "Now I'm in control." You'll feel convinced you can meet the challenge with energetic confidence. Isn't this exactly how you want to feel when meeting a challenge?

Exercise also guards against excess cortisol output and increases endorphin output. Endorphins are a natural drug produced in the brain. We teasingly say it's the most powerful legal drug on earth, and all you have to do is exercise, laugh, or touch someone to access it.

Exercise Intensity

Exercise is like a pension plan: The more you put in now, the more you'll have later. In the case of exercise, the more you do now, the more time and energy you'll have later to enjoy your pension plan.

Like socks, one exercise routine doesn't fit all. You need to tailor your exercise routine to your condition, age, and life roles.

Seriously out-of-shape couch potatoes get overstressed merely by taking the long hike down the hall to the refrigerator; such individuals need exercise desperately, but they must approach it with great caution to avoid serious consequences. You see, there is a training effect to being a couch potato, and these bodies have been trained for endurance sitting and have adapted to inactivity, so any movement is stressful.

The group most in danger of overdoing exercise includes men under 50 who, though athletic when younger, have not exercised much for ten years or more. These individuals often feel immune to the risks of suddenly becoming intensely active. They're not immune, however, as some grieving families discover. Get a medical checkup first, start slowly, and proceed with caution.

Researchers are now studying whether moderate exercise such as golfing with a hand-pulled cart, or leisurely 30-minute strolls offer any benefit. Many in the field say any exercise is certainly better than no exercise. But why stop there? This much is already clear: The average individual who goes out for at least moderately vigorous exercise will live much longer than someone who doesn't. Today's research strongly suggests you should exercise as frequently and as vigorously as you safely can if one of your goals is to prolong your highly functional years.

However, you must use common sense. I'm absolutely amazed at the way some businesspeople exercise here in Florida. I commend them for heading out to jog or cycle to maintain their vigor for work, but I condemn one thing some of these people do. Even in the summer when it's hot and humid, they don plastic jogging outfits or rain suits, thinking they will sweat more and burn more calories. But the skin can't breathe under these conditions. Sure, they'll sweat more because perspiration is the body's cooling system, but because the sweat can't evaporate from the skin to cool off, the heat builds up. Their bodies actually begins cooking. Those who exercise this way risk heat exhaustion, dehydration, and other serious consequences. And they run these risks for nothing because any weight lost will be regained when they quench their thirst.

Stay away from nonbreathable materials. Wear cotton clothing when exercising to facilitate evaporation to cool your body.

Beginning an Exercise Program

If you're a typical executive—overstressed mentally and emotionally, understressed physically—you're storing excess fat around the middle. For male executives this is usually on the stomach, and for female executives it is usually on the thighs, hips, and back of the arms. No matter where the fat settles, its excess weight gets hauled along every step you take, making movement more fatiguing and immobility more tempting. When you decide to take a stab at getting rid of some of your excess fat, you immediately hit snags on your way to svelte.

Beware of the two most common ways of failing to achieve greater stamina by increasing your exercise and decreasing your fat intake:

1. You lose interest because you don't see results right away. Results take time. Give yourself ample time to regain your former suppleness, muscle mass, and stamina. As you start your personal improvement project, make a careful inventory of your present condition. Record your weight, and don't check it again for three months. Instead, measure your waist, thigh, and other strategic points. Take a reading on your ratio of body fat to lean body mass (muscle) with skin-fold calipers. Note your resting heart beat by finding the pulse in your wrist. Count the beats for six seconds, add a zero to the result, and you have your heart beat rate for a minute. For more accuracy, count the beats for 15 seconds and multiply by 4. The more starting benchmarks you record, the more chances you'll have to encourage yourself by noting improvements.

2. You dive into strenuous exercise too fast, injure yourself, and have to quit "temporarily." Then you take months to get started again, or you never do. Increase your exercise level cautiously. Any injuries you might sustain should be small enough that you can continue to workout around them. For example, if you have sore ankles from running too soon, switch to swimming until your ankles feel okay again.

16 Ways to Increase the Fun of Exercise

Exercise will definitely improve your performance at work and with your family. In both vital areas of your life, you'll be more energetic, effective, and creative.

1. Exercise. It's an enormous power to extend and enhance your life. You can live longer with exercise. In the *New England*

Journal of Medicine (February 25, 1993), Ralph Paffenbarger, of Harvard University, published his study of 10,269 Harvard alumni (all men), whom he had tracked for 20 years. He discovered an interesting fact: Those who spent three hours a week in moderately vigorous activity had reduced their chances of dying from any cause during the 20-year period by 50 percent! For an individual to achieve such an exciting result, only moderately vigorous exercise is required. Playing tennis, brisk walking, swimming, low-impact video aerobics, cross-country skiing, or snowshoeing qualify. Running or vigorous cycling isn't required.

Paffenbarger identified four separate factors associated with lower rates of death from all causes among middle-aged and older men. The factors are: (1) engage in moderately vigorous sports activity, (2) stop smoking cigarettes, (3) maintain normal blood pressure, and (4) avoid obesity. Although Paffenbarger limited his study to men—perhaps to isolate a larger sample and make follow-up easier—these factors likely apply to women with equal force.

Paffenbarger's study is further supported by the 1996 Surgeon General's Report on Physical Activity and Health, which shows that exercise is as important to your overall health as it is for a smoker to quit smoking. These amazing findings should inspire you to enhance and extend your life by making some small changes in your present lifestyle. Nevertheless, some people will disregard this information for two common reasons:

A. *They choose not to believe Paffenbarger's study.* Since an additional 20 to 50 years of your life depend on your taking Paffenbarger seriously, spend a few hours looking up his study. (A good public library will have the article on microfilm.) Before you dismiss his conclusions out of hand, it makes sense to at least know how he reached them.

B. *They don't think the numbers apply to them.* They say, "Other people have heart attacks and cancer—I don't." Some splendid, warmhearted, and highly capable people seem oddly convinced that they are somehow immune to the perils of their death-accelerating lifestyles. Unfortunately, many of them stick to such lifestyles until the axe falls.

A friend of mine traveled this route. Woody was the hard-driving, chain-smoking sales manager of an auto parts distributor. He insisted, "If lung cancer hits me, that's the way it has to be. I'm not going to stop smoking."

As it happened, lung cancer missed him. He did stop smoking, though—after his first heart attack—not soon enough. His second heart attack a year later closed his file. A few small changes in his lifestyle would have given him a good shot at an additional 40 years of life. Woody was two weeks short of his 45th birthday when he died.

Exercise also contributes to two other factors in Paffenbarger's study: maintaining normal blood pressure and avoiding obesity. The last factor, stop smoking, simply requires you to make and act on a decision to put your personal survival ahead of the tobacco industry's profits.

Exercise will add years to your life and—through the added release of hormones such as endorphins—add life to your years. From two standpoints, job performance and longevity, it's vital to be moderately active. If you've been fighting it—making excuses, not finding time, or being resentful about its necessity—stop. Reconsider. This isn't like deciding whether to renew your subscription to *National Geographic*—it's a matter of life or death—literally. Make exercise an important priority in your routine.

2. Start easy. By starting easy, you avoid injury and, equally important, frustration. Trying to do too much too soon damages your self-esteem uselessly. You should feel great about embarking on a new adventure to rebuild your fitness and stamina. Avoid setting yourself up to feel like a loser because you can't meet the unnecessarily difficult demands you impose upon your unready body. Give yourself a break. Enjoy every improvement you make, no matter how small.

Never, ever, compare yourself to anyone else. In the great, ongoing tournament of self-improvement, your only opponent is your former, less fit, self.

3. Go for the fun things first. The first choice of many new exercisers is the stationary bicycle. It's available rain or shine, and you can read the paper, watch TV, or listen to tapes while you exercise. My personal favorite is the LifeCycle by Life

Fitness, Inc., because it's designed for interval training, and some models include a sensor for checking heart rate.

However, in good weather and where you have safe and convenient paths or lanes, most people find biking or inline skating in the fresh outdoors far more interesting. Hiking, or simply walking, is another happy choice for exercise beginners. Swimming, water-skiing, and other water sports can build your enthusiasm for exercise. If you haven't water-skied for several years, go easy your first day back on skis. In what seems like no more than a few minutes, you can overwork long-neglected muscles so much you'll be stiff and sore for a week.

4. Add variety. Variety beats boredom. Switching from one activity to another not only holds down boredom, but it's better for you because it exercises different muscles. For variety as well as overall strength-building, go for variety in all your exercises. Rather than following the exact same weight-lifting routine month after month, add new exercises and drop old ones. After training hard at his specialty for months, Roger Banister took off on a rock-climbing trip to Scotland. Then he came back just in time for a race and, without another training run, broke the four-minute mile for the first time in history. I believe the variety of his routine gave him the edge that he needed.

5. Challenge yourself with realistic goals. After you get into the swing of regular exercise, start setting realistic goals for yourself. Try for a little more only when you feel a little stronger. Push cautiously into the area of slight discomfort in physical stress.

Don't fall for the dangerous "No pain, no gain" misconception. Rhyme made those words stick, but do not confuse pain, which is a warning to your body that should be avoided, with the healthy "burn" exercisers feel by going a bit beyond their comfort zone. The burn—merely a slight discomfort—lets you know you've reached the level of stress that causes adaptation (increased endurance and muscle growth) during the recovery period of the day.

6. Exercise for yourself—not because your spouse, your boss, or even this book says you should. Set up your own rewards and goals for exercise and smarter eating. The greatest reward—a longer, more vibrant life—is automatic but tends to be undervalued, perhaps because we get our reward only one moment at a time. It's not like St. Peter comes along and says, "Okay, people, you've been eating and exercising right, so we're giving you an extra 20 years on Earth."

7. Exercise when your body will benefit most—in the late afternoon or early evening. You say you're a morning person who likes to "get the sweating out of the way first thing?" Sure, in the morning the air is fresh, traffic is light, and your mind is filled with the new day's exciting challenges and possibilities. However, if you're a desk worker whose only strenuous exercise is your daily workout, your body isn't ready for it in the morning. According to the research, the hours of late afternoon or early evening—4 p.m. to 7 p.m.—are the best hours to exercise for three reasons: (1) After work, exercise delivers a powerful recovery wave from the tensions of the day; (2) in the evening, your normal circadian rhythm provides a mix of chemical neurotransmitters far better suited to exercise than what's available in the morning; and (3) you're usually under less time pressure.

8. Walk or ride a bicycle at least part-way to work. If the distance involved and other conditions make it feasible, ease into it slowly. Check the route carefully by car first. Make sure you can travel on bike lanes or bike paths, with no dangerous intersections to cross or tight roads to negotiate. Then start with a portion of the route no further than you regularly bike—your first day biking to work is not the time to start endurance training on a bike.

Examine all the angles before you start biking to work. Where can you lock your bike and helmet? Where will you shower and change clothes? With a bike rack on your car, you can drive part-way, find a safe place to leave your car, and get on your bike to complete your journey. If you do this, make sure you can get a ride back to your car in case an unexpected storm hits.

9. Make a habit of climbing stairs instead of taking the elevator. Climbing all the way isn't realistic if your destination is on the 35th floor. In this case, take the elevator to the 32nd floor, run up three flights, and arrive emotionally and physically invigorated by a bit of exercise. For the more common trip, up just two or three floors, the stairs offer exercise with little or no loss in time. In many buildings, you'll save time running up the stairs, as opposed to waiting for an elevator. Many people find climbing stairs at work, instead of being lifted mechanically, makes a tremendous difference in their vitality.

10. Listen to audio books as you walk, run, jog, bike, rollerblade, pump iron, ride a stationary bicycle, or trot on a treadmill. Not everyone enjoys the solitude of biking or jogging alone with their thoughts. There's no longer any reason to dread the boredom of working out on machines or pounding down the road. Equip yourself with a belt-attachable cassette player so you can listen to audio-books and exercise your mind while you exercise your body. A word of caution: Make sure you can still hear what's going on around you while you have the earphones on. Otherwise you might get hit by a driver who thinks you can hear his vehicle motoring along.

11. Keep reinforcing why you exercise. Here's a sample affirmation: "I love working out and exercising because it makes me feel great. While I'm getting stronger, I'm also gaining a competitive edge over (enemies, rivals, or competitors) to boost my chances of (reaching a social or career goal). I love working out and exercising because I know I'll live longer and better, and I love it because it boosts my confidence and makes me feel good about myself."

12. Work out with a companion, but don't rely on him or her. Depending on someone else to show up for your workouts can easily prevent you from working out at all; still, many people find that when they work out with a dependable friend, they exercise more. Some find it better to organize a group of four to six people, so even if one or two people don't show up, there's still companionship. Do what works for you.

13. Treat yourself to the latest gear. You don't actually need expensive paraphernalia to exercise, but the plain fact of the matter is the gadgets, gear, and jazzy outfits make it a lot more fun for most people. When you're just starting your program and are maybe a trifle bulgy, you may not feel comfortable highlighting the shape you're in with tight workout clothing. If so, make wearing the latest, trendiest, and flashiest workout clothes one of your goals and rewards. In any case, go with whatever gets you to exercise.

14. Enter competitions and join health clubs. Competition is a powerful spur to train harder. Competition isn't only for the marathoners and triathletes; it's for everybody. Shorter races such as the 5K (five kilometers, slightly more than 3 miles) are held frequently. Tennis tournaments at country clubs or municipal parks often divide the competitors by ability level. If you look for it, you'll find a whole world of exciting, inspiring, health-building competition in one sport or another. No matter what your circumstances, you can find healthy competition in which you won't be seriously outclassed. The possibilities include supermarathons for paraplegics, senior and special Olympics, and guest races at ski resorts.

Health clubs not only offer a vast array of workout equipment, they also throw you in with people who are exercisers. Joining a health club can be inspiring and determination-building, or it can multiply your frustrations. Find what works for you and go with it.

15. Use an exercise band. In place of weights, use an exercise band. Several brands are on the market. Exercise bands do not replace the variety of strength-building machines available in gyms, but a band is convenient, can be used anywhere, and is ideal for starting an exercise program. It's also great for filling in the gaps when you can't get to a gym.

Exercise bands are inexpensive, versatile, light, and simple. Most slip into a pocket, purse, or briefcase, and are always ready for instant use, whether you need a quick exercise refresher or a long workout. Only your imagination limits the number of stretches and strength-building exercises you can perform with one.*

16. Park at the far end of the lot. When you drive to work, go shopping, or make sales calls, park in spaces far away from the entrance. Why drive through the entire parking lot searching for a space near the entrance when you could use an invigorating walk?

Select Programs to Improve Your Lean Body Mass-to-Fat Ratio

If you feel the need for local supervision and encouragement in your drive to enhance energy and performance, I urge

---

*Please contact LGE Sport Science at 1-800-543-7764 to obtain an exercise band with instruction manual by Pat Etcheberry, the world's top fitness trainer in golf and tennis.

you to avoid two kinds of programs: those that push you to buy most of your food from them, and those that don't put major emphasis on exercise. Such programs seem more concerned with profit than with their customers' health and weight.

Don't think in terms of weight loss. Focus on the ratio between lean body mass and body fat—the most important issue in improving health and boosting performance. Weight is simply an unreliable indicator of either health or performance potential. Losing weight without exercise eliminates more muscle tissue than fat.

If you are seriously overweight, find a local doctor who specializes in treating obesity. Get his or her approval and advice about how you go about exercising, which will be more stressful than if you were starting closer to your ideal weight.

If you aren't already a regular exerciser, get your doctor's approval before starting any exercise program. Once you've done so, find a convenient health club or gym where you feel comfortable. Use it three times a week for strength-building workouts. Many health clubs also provide facilities for aerobic exercise and endurance training. If your club can't help with the endurance element of your program, organize your routine around some activity you enjoy: tennis, racquetball, rollerblading, biking, hiking, walking, swimming, or whatever fits your schedule.

In making your choice of a health club, look for convenience and time-effectiveness, two vital elements in any successful program.

Getting a Grip on Your Body Image

We are surrounded by "model-thin" people in the media. I have worked with model-thin people who are still carrying too much fat, and, although they may look good on the outside, they are not necessarily healthy on the inside. Model-thin is not necessarily in.

Spot reducing and body contouring are exciting concepts to many of us. The problem is, the desired results don't occur, and more stress is created. However, exercise has a wonderful ability to reshape your self-image. In the first place, it will give you an attractive, more toned look, which is rightly prized. Regular exercisers tend to move more gracefully, carry themselves straighter, and project more energy.

People who participate in sports, particularly women, tend to appreciate their body shapes more than sedentary women do, whether or not they approach the model-thin curvaceousness society holds up as perfection. Part of this may stem from the fact that being tall or big is an advantage in some sports.

As noted by researchers, regular exercise also helps establish a positive family environment. Exercising together not only helps keep the family close, its members also have less time or inclination to indulge in activities harmful to health.

Your Rescue Mission: Save Your Own Arteries

Your body is very adaptable. If you've been active, you have a head start; if not, you may have some work to do. The body is designed to be active, but if you become sedentary, you automatically train your body to do nothing.

- Begin by setting goals you can reach. Start slowly and work your way into sports gradually. Just as you need to progressively work your way toward a higher level of activity over a period of weeks, you need to begin each exercise session by warming up for a few minutes.
- Schedule enough recovery after every exercise day, or follow an aerobic training day with a strength training day. The stress of exercise is the stimulus for growth, but you grow (get stronger or gain stamina) during your recovery time.
- Reverse the effects of poor nutrition and couch-potato syndrome and improve the quality of your life and health.

Chapter 8

NUTRITION AS RECOVERY

*"The majority of American men believe that
if they're not sick, they must be healthy."*
—Robert S. Ivker

Do you share the common belief that if you're not sick, you're healthy enough to perform at high levels at the office and with your family? Unfortunately, few people think in terms of setting health goals beyond hoping to avoid infectious diseases, accidents, and migraine headaches. This attitude precludes putting much effort into reaching the peak of vigorous vitality.

What Is Health?

Good health is not simply physical. Truly healthy people are physically, emotionally, and mentally strong, resilient, flexible—and powerfully responsive to the challenges and opportunities of life. In a word, they are tough. Being tough is far more than not being sick; toughness allows each individual who achieves it to maximize his or her potential.

You don't have to settle for merely being well and pain free; you can achieve glowing health and toughness and function at your ultimate performance potential. However, you can't reach those levels of glorious living and working without effort—or maintain them without sacrifice. It takes training to get there. Staying there means sacrificing the practices now weakening your health and interfering with high performance. If you are to reach your maximum potential, you need to get enough recovery in the form of sleep, relaxation, and fun; be physically active; stop smoking and abusing alcohol; and eat more of the right things.

Why Is Commitment to Intelligent Nutrition So Difficult?

From my traveling, working with groups, and talking to thousands of people in private consultations, I conclude that there are four reasons why commitment to nutrition is difficult:

1. Lack of a strategy to make (and keep) a commitment. This is the most common problem I encounter. For this reason, I will show you how to make the commitment and keep it.

2. The "I don't have time to eat well" copout. Anyone could use this excuse to avoid eating well. There are plenty of healthy take-out foods available, such as apples, bagels, and so on. Thousands of people eat well. Anyone who doesn't simply won't make the effort.

3. The "I just like foods that are bad for me" excuse. Every other kid on the block does, too. It's time to take control of your performance level and longevity expectation before bad food kills you in your prime.

4. The "I'm simply not hungry when I wake up" complaint. This negative message says your daily routine is out of balance. Your most serious needs probably are for more exercise and more sleep. Begin your move to a healthier lifestyle by eating a smaller dinner earlier in the evening so you'll sleep better and be hungry for breakfast when you wake up. This plan will give you the energy to become more active.

How Well Do You Fuel Your Body for High Performance?

What if you put great high octane fuel in your race car only on race day, but every other day you tried to make it perform on diesel fuel? What do you think of that as a plan to win races? Of course, it's an outline for disaster. If your race car would run at all, it certainly wouldn't deliver maximum performance on race days.

You face the same problem every day that it's to your advantage to perform well—more than likely this means every day of your working career. If you want to perform to your maximum potential, consider yourself a high performance Ferrari and fuel your system accordingly. Are you putting high octane or diesel fuel in your body?

Nutrition and the Ideal Performance State

What exactly is the Ideal Performance State (IPS)? The IPS is the most effective and reliable mental, emotional, and physical state for performing at your best. IPS is characterized by specific positive emotions of being calm, confident, relaxed, energized, fun-loving, and fulfilled. Being able to access this state on demand is an essential characteristic of successful performers.

In sports, the idea of being "in the zone" is well known. In business it is known as being "on a roll." Not only is it possible to achieve that state in business and in life, reaching your highest potential depends on doing so.

I believe (and research supports this belief) that what and when we eat can powerfully affect our mental state. If so, then two things are vitally important: (1) We are in almost total control of our performance state, and (2) nutrition may be one of the most crucial factors in high-performance business today.

In 20 years of training athletes, I have run across many who felt they were doing the right things nutritionally. Their wake-up call came after a nutritional profile compared their daily food consumption with their height, weight, age, gender, and activity level.

I have worked with elite athletes whose self-images were ones of being fat when their body fat percentage actually was close to ideal, whose fat intake was too high, who tried fad diets and fad foods, who didn't eat enough calories, who had vitamin and mineral deficiencies, who ate too many sweets, who didn't replace fluids well, and a few athletes who would eat anything if they thought it would give them a competitive edge.

These were individuals at the top of their sports, but once they realized these nutritional shortcomings, they raised their performances even higher. Some were even shocked at the limitations they had placed on themselves through subpar nutrition.

Physiologically and psychologically, poor nutrition can be a major limiting factor in sports. The same is true in business and life. Poor nutrition severely weakens your ability to access the Ideal Performance State.

We are creatures of emotion! If you don't believe it, think about how many times in life you have been irritable. How many times have you been happy? Sad? Fatigued? Bored? Annoyed?

Out of sorts? Now the fun begins. In each of these feelings, evaluate how well you performed, whether at work or with your family. I bet that you were the best performer when you felt good, and not when negative feelings were present.

Perform on Demand

When we examine the mega-performers in business today, we find they are readily able to access the positive emotions responsible for high performance. In the Anti-Diet program, I call that ability *Performance on Demand.*

Do you think Michael Eisner always gets enough sleep before going to work? Do you think Bill Gates never gets stuck in traffic before going to a big meeting? Do you believe Estee Lauder, directing a multibillion-dollar enterprise, ever worked without stress? To these great executives, the fact that they did not sleep well at night, were stuck in traffic, arrived late for a meeting, or even ate something that disagreed with their stomach had nothing to do with pulling off a great performance. Early in their careers, they all learned one of the cruelest and coldest facts about corporate life: No one cares whether you slept last night or had a fight with your spouse this morning— you still have to perform, and perform well.

Was this ability to perform on demand a learned skill? I find that it is 100 percent learned. Regardless of the competitive arena—business, sports, or life—the mega-performers learn how to access the Ideal Performance State whenever and wherever they need it. In fact, today we know that possessing talent and skill is not enough: You must learn how to bring the full force of all your talents and skills to life when you need them.

Psychological studies have shown that success in business or sports is connected more to your ability to access the Ideal Performance State than it is to talent or skill. Because with IPS you get balance, perspective, enjoyment, poise, calmness, positive energy, and the passion to fight the battle.

Who's Got It? How Do I Get It?

The key to accessing the IPS emotions on demand is toughness training. Toughness is the ability to consistently perform toward the upper range of your talent and skill. Along with my partners, Jim Loehr and Pat Etcheberry, I have devoted the last 20 years to studying and understanding how performers in business and sports get tougher.

We have found that everyone in a competitive arena is subjected to world-class stress from time to time. The one common factor that separates the great performers from good or average performers is that great performers know how to balance stress and recovery so well that they get world-class recovery that matches their world-class stress.

What Is Recovery?

If stress is the expenditure of energy, then recovery is the recapturing of energy—literally, recharging your batteries. Just as there is an Ideal Performance State, there is an Ideal Recovery State (IRS). As an aside, this may be the only time your life when the initials IRS are positive.

The most powerful and essential mechanism of recovery is sound sleep of adequate duration. Nutrition, including drinking enough water, is next in importance.

For people whose work is primarily mental, getting enough exercise to maintain stamina is the third most important mechanism of recovery. To the mentally and emotionally overtrained executive, physical exercise provides an essential release from stress that can be obtained in no other way. By solving the relatively minor problems connected with building adequate exercise breaks into their daily routines, motivated executives can gain a formidable competitive edge over the usual couch potato opposition.

Having fun—enjoying each day to the utmost whether at work or at play—is the fourth most powerful mechanism of recovery. The ability to laugh, to find fun in what you do, is a priceless asset.

So powerful is laughter that it can extend your ability—although only briefly—to carry on without adequate food or rest, especially in extreme situations. Laughter is nature's own way of giving us more flexibility with the other basic recovery mechanisms. In fact, it is the only nonharmful way to do this.

The most common drugs used to extend people's ability to

perform without adequate rest or food, or as substitutes for adequate enjoyment in one's life—caffeine, nicotine, and alcohol—are legal. But the consequences of their abuse are too well documented to require much comment here. I will only say that their extensive use indicates a seriously out-of-balance lifestyle.

Without question, the foods you eat influence your brain chemistry, performance, mood, and alertness. When you eat and how you feel when you eat are also important. Thus, in most instances you are in control of setting your emotional state.

The Corporate Athlete's Nutritional Needs

Your nutritional recovery needs should look like this at most meals:

2 servings	complex carbohydrates
1-2 servings	protein
.5 -1 serving	fat

All of us have seen ratios like these (often in the form of percentages) for years, but what do they mean? How do you know if what you're now eating comes close? The key is that you maintain a well-balanced nutritional program so you have the right mix of protein, carbohydrates, and fat. But these numbers will help:

1 gram of protein	= 4 calories
1 gram of carbohydrate	= 4 calories
1 gram of fat	= 9 calories
1 gram of alcohol	= 7 calories

It doesn't take a mental giant to see that you can eat twice as much protein and carbohydrate as fat. In fact, the key to great nutrition is limiting your fat intake.

Let's assume that you need 2,000 calories a day. (Some people need a little less and some a little more depending on how active they are and what their body composition is.) What we're aiming for then is—

1/2 of your intake is carbohydrates= 1,000 calories (divided by 4)=250 grams

1/4 to 1/3 of your intake is protein = 600 calories (divided by 4) = 150 grams

1/6 to 1/4 of your intake is fat = 400 calories (divided by 9) = 44.4 grams

Nutrition as Recovery

How do you regard the food you eat? Primarily as a source of pleasure? As a reward? As solace when you're unhappy? As a source of emotional satisfaction in hostile or unprofitable situations? As a means of recovering not only expended energy but also expended minerals and vitamins?

In the list of mechanisms of recovery, nutrition is rated second behind sleep. For maximum performance, take care of your recovery needs first. That is, eat foods and consume liquids that enable you to recover the nutrients you have expended since your last refueling. For best results, make every pit stop for fuel as enjoyable as possible, but don't lose sight of your primary purpose: to replenish what you've expended.

The Two Most Important—and Most Overlooked—Nutrients!

Curiously, most of us force our bodies to exist on minimum intakes of our two most pressing needs: oxygen and water. It can be argued that water is our most important nutrient, except that it isn't a nutrient in the sense most people understand the word. Neither is oxygen commonly thought of as a nutrient, yet it's the most demanding need our bodies have. Without oxygen, life is measured in seconds; without water, in days; without food, in weeks.

Oxygen. Few people practice deep breathing, even though doing so consumes no time at all, requires little effort, and pays big dividends in increased energy. It can be done while you are sitting, standing, walking, or lying down. You can breathe deeply at odd moments when occupied by necessary but low-intensity things like dressing, riding to work, and waiting for an elevator door to open.

Practice deep breathing frequently during the day. Inhale, on a slow count of four, all the air you can, and then exhale on a slow count of eight. Do this ten times as soon as you wake up in the morning. You'll find that it clears the morning fog quickly.

Water. Our bodies are made mostly of water, which we constantly use in a number of ways, of which perspiration and excretion are merely the most obvious. You must replenish your water-based system frequently by drinking 64 ounces (eight glasses) of water every day. Sodas don't count. Coffee and tea are diuretics; they cause you to lose more water. Rather than helping you meet your body's daily water requirement, coffee and tea have the opposite effect.

Only about nine percent of the professionals in corporate America drink more than seven glasses of water a day. The consumption of water is critical for both body and cerebral functions.

The biggest complaint I get is, "Wait a minute, I'll be going to the bathroom all day." My answer is, "That's okay, it won't take long."

Even if you keep a glass of water on your bedside table, you're still somewhat dehydrated when you wake up after a good night's sleep. Many of us have trained our bodies to accept this situation, and in any case, the thirst feeling is not a reliable indicator of mild dehydration.

As soon as you get up, drink a full 8-ounce glass of cool water. It's so easy, and it does so much to prime your body to shift into high gear. There's another advantage to drinking a glass of water first thing in the morning: It gets you off to a flying start toward fulfilling your body's need for eight glasses a day. If you shortchange your body on water; you shortchange yourself on stamina.

Keep in mind that our bodies are over half water. It's constantly being consumed in countless ways, among them digestion, body cooling, blood replacement, elimination of wastes, and lubrication of the joints. In fact, all of our cell processes and organ functions depend on water. If you force your body to function without giving it enough water, it can't perform to its highest potential.

The Issue of Thirst

Can you dehydrate just living a normal day? Absolutely. Although your water loss isn't as noticeable as that of a sweaty athlete, you're losing water constantly through a variety of normal body processes—you perspire to some degree even in an air-conditioned building. But even without that, you lose water constantly through the pores of your skin. Your body also uses water for numerous lubrication, digestion, elimination, and replacement activities that are constantly going on. In fact, it's not practical to try to list all the body's needs for water; suffice it to say that nothing works without water.

Even though it's so vital to our very existence, we tend to ignore our water needs until, going without, we become quite uncomfortable. Don't take feeling thirsty merely as a signal that you need a drink of water right now; take it as a signal that your water replacement habits need some serious work. You should never get really thirsty.

Remember that you can easily satisfy your thirst before your body's needs for water are satisfied. Schedule your water intake; don't merely react to a thirsty feeling.

Coffee and tea are not considered alternatives to water because their diuretic action makes you lose more water than you gain by drinking them. Many soft drinks also contain caffeine, and between the diuretic effect and the stress put on your system to cope with their sugar content, it's questionable whether you have a net gain of moisture from drinking one.

Alcohol is even more of a diuretic, since it must be broken down by the liver and kidneys—a process that consumes considerable amounts of water. If the stomach doesn't have water available, your kidneys will pull it out of your body's cells. The "cotton mouth" you get the morning after the big party is due to dehydration. It's not a joking matter when you consider that you've just struck a blow to the health of every cell in your body.

For satisfying your body's unceasing need for water, nothing is better than just plain water, preferably cool rather than ice-cold.

How do you know if you're drinking enough water? You'll know you're drinking enough if you drink eight glasses a day.

Scheduling Nutrition as Recovery

In the military you're not allowed to skip breakfast—that would get you 100 push-ups. You are not allowed to skip lunch, either. There's a method behind this apparently blind authoritarianism: The military knows that soldiers who skip breakfast or lunch perform below expectations—if they don't poop out completely.

But why, then, do we in business so often skip breakfast or lunch? And often, when we eat lunch, we're in such a hurry that we try to scarf it down in the fewest bites possible.

You never see animals skip a meal, or eat a meal so quickly that gastrointestinal distress erupts. We are members of the animal kingdom—biological organisms. And as such we must nourish our animal selves, not a disembodied set of brain waves soaring in cyberspace. *Don't just fit meals in. Schedule your meals as mechanisms of recovery.* It's that crucial!

Chapter 9

THE CORPORATE ATHLETE'S POWERBUILDING RECOVERY REGIME

*"I know of no businessman who said on his deathbed,
'Aw, shucks, I wish I'd spent more time at the office.'"*
—Will Rogers

Like many executives, you've given your all to your corporate career. Work comes first. You believe it's absolutely necessary to look at things that way if you are to stay on top of the demands of your position. Shoulder to the wheel, nose to the grindstone, gets the job done.

Well, maybe not. Several studies of top executives have shown that they tend to be heavily involved with their families and communities. This is not something that starts after they've reached the top; they follow this pattern their entire careers. Looking closer at highly successful people, we find that as a group they tend to be relaxed, and they enjoy their work.

"Sure," you say, "who wouldn't, with all their perks?" But that doesn't explain how they managed to have fun and live a full non-business life *while* they climbed the ladder to success.

Have Fun at What You Do

It's easy to love what you do. Many people love their work, but that's vastly different from having fun at what you do. Being able to find or create fun in your work ranks with physical toughening, healthy nutrition, and other recovery mechanisms for emotional and mental toughening. Without fun, achieving high velocity in your life and career is possible but risky, and likely to be short-lived, because laughter is the strongest defense against excessive mental stress.

Humor is the mother of creativity (the father is perspiration), and as such it can play a powerful role in building profits. In countless other indirect ways, humor benefits the bottom line. I don't suggest that horseplay or dangerous practical jokes should be tolerated, but these are a far cry from relaxed fun-seeking at work. Give high priority to developing and encouraging humor and gentle jokes that demean or offend no one. Using the release of laughter as frequently as possible is the best alertness extender imaginable.

To develop greater stamina for business, first accept the fact that it's built on many pilings:
• Toughen yourself physically.
• Toughen yourself mentally.
• Toughen yourself emotionally.
• Build more laughter into your life.
• Make sure your recovery balances your stress.
• Eat for stamina, high performance, and health.

Six Keys to Better Health and Higher Performance

Just as all six cylinders must be firing for a V-6 engine to reach full power, it takes all six of these keys to unlock your ultimate level of health and performance:

1. Get going on regular workouts. At the minimum, you should exercise to reach your training heart rate and maintain it for 30 minutes three times a week. Research shows that three 10-minute training sessions per day confer about the same cardiovascular benefits as a single 30-minute workout. This gives you greater flexibility in organizing your workouts.

Vary your exercise method to keep it interesting. A hard-fought tennis match may give you a terrific workout along with being lots of fun. A game of basketball or a martial arts class can have the same effect. Relying on sports to provide some of your regular workouts inspires you to train yourself into better shape—and have fun doing it.

2. Power your thoughts. During most of our waking moments, a stream of consciousness keeps running through our heads with a torrent of about 50,000 thoughts a day. This self-talk is difficult to discipline except in deep meditation. It starts in childhood and continues throughout our adult life. As a result, we tend to let it run on automatic, like our breathing, but this basic carelessness poses enormous dangers.

Left to themselves, our thoughts fall back on our deepest survival instincts, which tend to be negative and overly protective of our delicate egos. You can change this by consciously directing your self-talk with affirmations. Make seizing full, conscious control of your self-talk a major part of your toughening effort, and you'll speed your progress enormously. Write your positive affirmations down and review them at least twice a day. Start with, "I can do it."

People stuck on negative thoughts tend to dismiss the whole concept of paying close attention to nutrition and exercise as useless, unfair, and imposing. With such a negative automatic setting, we are not likely to seize or even see opportunities for growth.

Switching our automatic setting to positive thoughts fills us with hope and gives us feelings of worthiness and success. Because we are what we think about all day long, it's vital to power our thoughts positively. We will then see more challenges and fewer lost causes.

The vital thing to understand about your self-talk is this: You can take complete control of it.

3. Manage your heart rate. Heart rate management and zone training are important aspects of a workout. Check your heart rate while you're exercising. Take your pulse for a count of six and add a zero to get heart rate per minute. This method gives close enough results if you don't need frequent monitoring because of a medical condition. As you check your pulse, tune in, and learn how it feels to be in your target exercise zone.

To calculate your target zone, subtract your age from 220 to get your theoretical maximum heart rate. If your exercise goal is weight loss, take 60 percent for the lower limit and 70 percent for the higher and oscillate between those limits. If general cardiovascular fitness is your primary goal, oscillate between 70 and 85 percent of your maximum.

Keep an eye on your heart rate. Overtraining will slow—not speed—results.

4. Capitalize on humor. For recovery, humor is serious business. Laughter eases the mind, relieves stress, and strengthens your immune system. Your sense of humor deserves high priority. It can be a valuable self-renewing resource. Sarcastic humor and mean or sick jokes can plant undying hatreds. On the other hand, gentle humor, and especially jokes pointed at yourself or at your own expense, can be tools of great power to persuade, ease tension, open doors, and smooth the way in any negotiation. For the sake of your immune system and your career success, lose no opportunity to develop your ability to employ gentle humor and to feel a pervasive spirit of fun in all you do.

5. Eat smarter. Reduce the amount of total fat, but especially saturated fat, in your diet. Keep your intake of dietary cholesterol low to moderate, get enough protein, and make carbohydrates your main source of energy. Never skip breakfast, and make sure you eat several small meals a day with plenty of fruit and fresh vegetables. Take a multivitamin supplement as your insurance policy and drink plenty of water.

6. Sharpen your competitive edge. It's amazing in today's competitive business environment that most corporate executives don't eat to empower their minds, boost their energy, and increase their productivity. Their most important consideration in their decisions about what, where, and when to eat is convenience—the quick grab at sustenance-on-the-run. All too often the vital health considerations of fat avoidance, nutritional needs, and energizing values don't enter into the decision.

The second factor for many is taste, largely determined by habit. Unfortunately for their performance and longevity needs, most executives have food preferences that in at least one basic way parallel those of the general population: They love fat-heavy foods.

Taste and convenience are deciding factors in many executive meals, especially when time is tight. When the situation calls for a more leisurely business meal, usually the primary difference from a nutritional standpoint is that more calories are consumed. More time could easily lead to better food choices, but the opposite often occurs. Fat-laden entrees, fat-heavy sauces and dressings, rich desserts, and empty calories from drinks are frequent features of leisurely business meals.

The eating habits and lifestyles of most executives will change slowly—if at all—in the coming decades. This gloomy forecast for executive health has its bright side for the wise individual: You can get tougher while most people get weaker.

Commit to boosting your energy and mental acuity through better eating habits and by toughening yourself mentally, physically, and emotionally. You'll gain an important competitive edge over everybody who continues to grow heavier and softer while you're becoming leaner and stronger, more confident and quicker. In every area in which you compete, that edge will pay dividends.

The Pre-Challenge Meal

Especially important is the pre-challenge meal—what you eat before making a crucial sales presentation, giving a speech, or entering into an important negotiation. Depending on what you select, that meal can enable you to reach IPS, or it may prevent you from doing so. However, the pre-challenge meal works best as high-performance fuel when poured into a body long nourished wisely and well. The pre-challenge meal isn't a miracle cleansing agent any more than a tankful of high-octane fuel will clear a clogged engine on race day.

A diet that enables a great athlete to perform at a very high level is the same kind of diet that you, as a Corporate Athlete, should eat to stay healthy and to perform at a very high level in business and in life. This is what you should strive for.

By your own perception, how healthy is your diet? I often ask audiences to rate their diets on a scale from one to ten—ten being very healthy, one being very unhealthy. On the average, half of them give their own diets a six or under.

Probably, in your perception, your diet will fall somewhere in the middle between healthy and unhealthy. So you likely know you could eat better.

If you need a 2,000-calorie diet, you should not exceed 50 grams of fat on the average day. Your fat intake should chiefly consist of polyunsaturated and monounsaturated fats; minimize your intake of saturated fat (the kind you get from meat, egg yolks, butter, most desserts, creams, and so forth). If you stay under 50 grams most of the time, you can enjoy yourself without diet worries on special occasions.

If you have a Danish (24 grams of fat) in the morning, you're already half-way to your fat allotment. One croissant delivers 12 grams of fat, which amounts to 24 percent of your total daily limit. A four-ounce sirloin steak hits you with 21 grams of fat—all of it saturated. That's close to half your allotment.

On the other hand, an apple has no fat; an orange has only two-tenths of a gram of fat, and it's polyunsaturated. In other words, you'd have to eat over 220 oranges a day to reach your fat allotment from that source alone.

How to Eat When You Need to Perform at Your Best

Here are 10 basic guidelines:

1. Start developing your best pre-event meal long before the need. The important thing is what works for you. So find out through trial and error well before your gigantic, once-in-a-lifetime, do-or-die event. In particular, if you drink coffee or tea, find out what those stimulants do for you. Keep in mind that the effect you experience in low-tension situations will probably be magnified when tension is high.

2. Eat smart for at least 24 hours before a big event. Don't fall into the trap of thinking you can be careless about eating right up to show time, and then fix it all with a "magic bullet" meal. It doesn't work that way. To ensure maximum performance, come to your pre-event meal with your blood sugar holding steady. That means eating small, sensible meals five or six times a day in the week preceding the event.

3. Never eat a big pre-event meal. Big meals burden your body and blood supply with a heavy digestive demand that reduces your alertness and saps your energy.

4. Avoid alcohol. Alcohol is a powerful drug whose power to impair judgment and reduce alertness, even when consumed in small quantities, has been well-documented. Alcohol's effect on you is impossible to predict with certainty in the context of your performance at an important event. One little drink taken for whatever reason will often have the opposite effect of what you intend. *5. Avoid high-fat foods.* If you want to protect your performance potential, avoid fat-heavy foods before an event. Fatty foods linger in the stomach, providing little energy, and they demand so much digestive effort that your alertness may be reduced.

6. For an energizing effect, eat a light, low-fat meal that's no more than half carbohydrate, with protein making up the balance. This will increase the supply of endorphins in your brain, making it easier for you to access the Ideal Performance State, with all its attendant feelings of confidence and challenge.

7. Want to boost your alertness? Eat more protein. When you need to "get up" and want to boost your alertness, eat protein. If mood control isn't your main concern, eat for sustained energy. For an event you expect will go on for a long time, increase the carbohydrate portion of your pre-performance meal. For shorter performances, increase the protein. If hot temperatures are expected, eat a little less; if you anticipate cold, eat a little more. However, don't let a hot day keep you from fortifying your body with at least a minimum of sustainable energy.

8. Nervous? For a calming effect, eat a meal that is purely carbohydrate (no protein), if possible. Eating only carbohydrates will send more trytophan to the brain, where it will increase the supply of serotonin, a natural calming chemical. Eating even a small amount of protein blocks the calming effect.

9. Your best pre-event meal includes foods that you enjoy. As long as it's not loaded with fat or calories, be generous to yourself. Enjoy a favorite food before you perform. Eating what you like can have a tremendous positive effect.

10. Foods are like drugs—they can powerfully influence your mood. You'll find that your best pre-event meal can set you up to give your best performance, add to your confidence, and keep you alert and energetic. The rest is up to you.

The Corporate Costs of Poor Health

What does the explosion of obesity do to the outlook for medical plans? At every company, medical costs will escalate in the coming decades. This is certain to happen if each generation continues to get fat at an earlier age. It's our future unless the lifestyles of Americans take a small but vital turn toward better nutrition and more exercise.

Every corporation's executives have the wonderful opportunity and solemn duty not only to save themselves and their immediate families from succumbing to the obesity epidemic, but also to lead their employees and families in the direction of greater health and stamina. Beyond the altruistic element of this endeavor, there are solid, bottom-line reasons for driving hard to achieve it: sharply reduced absenteeism, enormous savings in medical costs, and vast economies achieved by having a healthier, more experienced and loyal work force capable of staying on the job year after year.

A vigorous, sustained program to encourage (not force) healthier lifestyles among the workforce, demonstrates—as few other policies can—management's genuine interest in employee welfare. Increased loyalty and internal goodwill naturally follow, along with important benefits in employee attitude and performance. I know it works and that it achieves splendid results because I have seen it happen in many companies.

However, no such results accrue when the program consists of nothing more than memos posted on the bulletin board and a few pep talks.

The 8-Phase Campaign to Boost Employee Productivity and Loyalty

Here's a practical program to boost employee productivity and loyalty. When it's fully implemented, it can make an enormous difference in the job performance of your entire work force:

1. *Top-level commitment must be strong enough to provide meaningful encouragement and incentives.* No substantial or permanent improvement in corporate culture, performance, and profitability will occur without such top-level support.

2. *Management must communicate what changes it hopes employees will make in their personal lifestyles.* This has to be done in a manner that will get them enthused about improving their health. Trainers and coaches can assist.

3. *Recognize and reward healthy lifestyles.* Since lifestyle quality controls performance, let it be known that it will be an important consideration in making promotions. Identify employees who already have healthy lifestyles, and those who make significant progress in improving their way of life, and recognize them in the newsletter and with perks.

4. Require the vendors who supply the food and drinks for vending macjines to include healthy, low-fat foods instead of candy, potato chips, and other high-fat snacks that tend to push some of your people toward poor cognitive performance and even early heart attacks.

Employee dissatisfaction with these changes can be minimized by first convincing everyone of its personal importance to them, and also by making the change over time. I recommend the following healthful snacks for vending machines:

- Fat-free pretzels.
- Fig newtons.
- Apples, bananas, and other fruits, along with vegetables and salads if your machines are serviced daily or if your facility has an employee cafeteria where fresh fruit can be offered.
- Canned fruit juices (but not sugar-added fruit drinks).
- Turkey sandwiches with lettuce and tomato on rye bread.
- Packaged raisins.
- Peanuts (though high in fat, peanuts are high in nutrients).
- Cinnamon raisin bagels (the flavor deters the need for cream cheese).
- Tuna sandwiches on whole-wheat bread.
- Grilled chicken breast sandwiches on multi-grain bread.

5. Eliminate the term "coffee break" from the human resources vocabulary. Use "recovery break" instead. Gradually reduce the accessibility and convenience of coffee in step with the progress of your educational program. Offer a variety of pure fruit juices and caffeine-free brands of soft drinks instead.

6. Prohibit smoking in all work areas and eliminate the sale of tobacco products.

7. Provide in-plant exercise facilities and make them available during work hours. Encourage their use to provide recovery waves that will permit employees in mentally and emotionally stressful positions (boring, repetitive work is emotionally stressful) to maintain their performance at peak levels throughout the workday.

8. *Encourage work groups* to begin their shifts with a routine of stretches and calisthenics.

Chapter 10

WANT TO CHANGE YOUR PHYSICAL APPEARANCE?

"Changing fitness appears to be at least as important as changing cholesterol level, blood pressure, body mass index, and smoking."
—Steven N. Blair

I often wonder what it will take to get Americans to change their eating and exercising habits. Maybe air travel should be charged by the pound. Or restaurants could refuse to serve anyone who has had too much to eat. The Internal Revenue Service could add a body fat tax table—taxing for every percent of body fat that exceeds the ideal. Then people who choose a high-fat diet would run up their tax bills instead of the country's medical costs.

On August 14, 1995, *USA Today* reported the goals that Americans said would motivate them to diet if they were overweight.

To be healthier . . . . 67 percent
To look better . . . . 21 percent
For a better love life . . . . 6 percent
To get a better job . . . . 3 percent
Don't know . . . . 3 percent

I know a few more reasons:
• To boost your stamina and health.
• To raise your performance level.
• To gain a better attitude, both at work and in your private life.

Time magazine called it "the decade's secret scandal," referring to the fact that instead of becoming more healthy in the health-conscious 1980s, "Americans actually plumped out." The article went on to discuss a long-term study by the Federal Center for Disease Control and Prevention. It revealed that the ratio of seriously overweight Americans, after holding steady for 20 years at about 25 percent of the population, shot up to 33 percent of the population during the '80s. This more than 30 percent increase for the entire nation in just ten years puts enormous numbers of people—over 80 million of them—at sharply increased health risk. Heart disease, gout, stroke, diabetes, hypertension, arthritis, and some types of cancer are among the degenerative diseases ignited or speeded by obesity.

Tremendous strides in medical technology, nutritional research, and exercise research during those years promised substantial increases in longevity. This expectation, torpedoed by junk food and fast food, sank without a trace in an ocean of fat.

Let's look at it this way: If you have stored more body fat under your skin than you need, it didn't just show up one morning. If you have spent several years drifting into a poor state of health, expect observable changes to take time. When those changes become obvious, you'll find them deeply satisfying and of great inspirational value in helping you continue your trip back to fitness, slenderness, and glowing health.

If you're serious about taking the trip to slenderness, stamina, and superb performance, please accept this fact: Dieting without exercise won't do it. Consider the following two examples: Solely by reducing his caloric intake, a 200-pound man with 23 percent fat loses 10 pounds. As a result, his body fat percentage rises significantly because much of his weight loss comes from lost muscle tissue. A 150-pound woman with 30 percent fat loses 10 pounds without exercising, sees her body fat percentage rise about a point, and wonders why she feels fatter and less fit.

How do you change your appearance through Anti-Dieting? Let's first agree that it won't happen before sun-up tomorrow. Whatever you want to change took some time to manifest itself, and it will take some time to reverse.

I assume what you want to change about your appearance has to do with having too high a ratio of fat to lean body mass. You'd like to look leaner, right?

To Look Like a Greek God or Goddess, Eat Like a Greek

On the Greek island of Crete, people kept to the traditional Mediterranean diet well into the 1960s. They ate heaps of fruits, grains, and vegetables laced with olive oil and some fish and poultry—but they ate very little red meat. They used so much olive oil that fat provided 40 percent of their calories. Americans are dying like flies on diets averaging the same 40 percent of calories from fat, but the Cretan death rate from coronary heart disease was only 5 percent of ours. In the middle of this century, Cretans and other Greeks were living longer than any other population in the world. As more and more of them abandoned the traditional Mediterranean diet in the succeeding decades, their death rates have risen significantly.

The Heart-Saving Mediterranean Diet

What did the long-lived Cretans and Greeks traditionally eat? Daily, they ate pasta, rice and other grains, breads, potatoes, a variety of vegetables and fruits, beans and other legumes, nuts, olive oil, cheese, and yogurt. A few times each week they ate fish, poultry, eggs, and sweets. Only a few times a month did they eat red meat.

In the 1960s, many Cretans were still farmers who burned much of the fat they consumed through hard labor. Another key element in producing the healthy effects of Mediterranean lifestyles was the absence of butter and mayonnaise with their high content of saturated fats. The olive oil, used instead, is rich in monounsaturated fats, which research points to as the healthiest kind of fat.

If the strong taste of olive oil is a problem, canola oil is a good substitute, since it contains even less saturated fat than olive oil and has more omega-3 fat.

In 1960 researchers learned the Mediterranean diet had slashed the rate of heart disease among Mediterranean peoples in half, as compared to their predicted rate based on their cholesterol level. That this is primarily due to the diet was proven by a recent French study of 600 heart-attack survivors. Half of them followed the Mediterranean diet; the other half ate the diet recommended by the U.S. Government and the American

Heart Association. After two years, the Mediterranean group had only 8 new heart attacks compared to 33 in the other group.

Slimming Down May Be Easier Than You Think

Many people are surprised to learn they can become leaner without feeling hungry or taking pills. A noticeable change can be achieved quickly.

Consider the case of Connie Lassoon, a young woman who came in to my office for consultation while I was writing this book. Connie was feeling rather desperate—for good reason. At 25 she weighed about 275 pounds although she was only 5 feet 3 inches tall. She had no self-esteem and no social life, and she believed her weight was a serious problem at work.

Before she came in she logged her food and drink intake for two days. Her diet proved interesting. For example, one day she had six large cheese raviolis with tomato sauce, 4 ounces of taco chips, 40 ounces of orange juice, 5 ounces of cheese-filled crackers, and 3 ounces of milk chocolate.

Most people might think the quantity of food is quite low. But when we analyzed that day, it came to almost 3,600 calories. She had consumed 112 grams of protein, 459 grams of carbohydrates, and the killer: 142 grams of fat.

To explain why I call 142 grams of fat, "the killer," let's take a close look at what eating so much fat a day does to the body. Since most of us are more familiar with the English ounce and pound system, a gram is a nebulous quantity. It doesn't help much to know there are a thousand of them in a 2.2 pound kilogram. A gram is only one-thousandth of 2.2 pounds. That converts to .035 ounce, or 1/28th of an ounce.

Still doesn't sound like much? Then consider this: If this young woman averages eating 142 grams of fat a day, she takes in 51,830 grams of dietary fat a year, or 116 pounds of the stuff. She doesn't burn much of it off because she's an inactive heavy eater, and the protein and carbohydrate elements of her food consumption easily take care of her daily requirements. Under these circumstances the body can convert much of the dietary fat into storable body fat. It may not occur exactly like this, but her story serves as a prime example because Connie has the potential to put on up to nine pounds a month! Yes, we're talking killer.

The second day was a little better. She had two cups of spaghetti noodles and one cup of spaghetti marinara sauce with mushrooms. For lunch she had a roast beef sandwich with pro- volone cheese and 5 tablespoons of mayonnaise. She also had 3 ounces of onion rings. Later in the day for a snack she had 2 ounces of pretzels, 1.5 ounces of milk chocolate, and a little Jell-O, and for dinner she had four fish sticks. That day was 2,500 calories with 126 grams of fat.

I then asked Connie what she might like to eat. She men- tioned bananas, strawberries, orange juice, pasta, chicken and such. As she talked, I entered her list in my computer and print- ed out what she might enjoy eating. At this point, I hadn't ana- lyzed my recommendations.

For example, in one day she could have 3 bananas, 1 cup of strawberries, 16 ounces of orange juice, a cup of spaghetti with 1/2 cup of marinara sauce, 1 skinless chicken breast, 3 ripe tomatoes, 1 cup sweet potatoes, 1 cup seedless grapes, 4 ounces of fat-free pretzels, and 16 ounces of skimmed milk.

Her first response before I analyzed it was, "That's impos- sible! I can't eat that much food!"

Then I analyzed it. The results astounded her. She saw the calories were 1,947. She thought it was incredible; she had imagined what I said she could have would have been way over what she had been eating before. By eating the more than ample diet I suggested, her fat intake would be a mere 20 grams for the entire day—well under an ounce and, more importantly, well under the amount her body had adapted to, so none would be stored as fat. In fact, with an intake of only 20 grams of fat a day—and with a modest increase in exercise— her body would draw on its ample supply of stored fat. In other words, she'd start losing weight. This young woman is well on the road to big changes in her life simply by identifying the fat content of foods when she wants to eat.

The "Oh, Woe Is Me" Syndrome

One problem Connie had I call the "Oh, woe is me" syn- drome. Every time she felt sorry for herself, got angry, or was overwhelmed by other negative feelings, Connie headed for the refrigerator. Since her refrigerator only held calorically dense foods with low nutrition values, she ate high-fat stuff that immediately took a long-term lease inside her skin.

By giving Connie alternative food choices she liked, she realized that even when she goes through an "Oh, woe is me" episode, she has healthful alternatives. She can eat almost twice as much food and still have fewer calories and much less fat.

In one instance I simply compared mayonnaise to mustard. Connie said she absolutely loved mayonnaise—putting away five tablespoons of mayonnaise in one day hadn't been unusual.

On the computer we found that 5 tablespoons of mayonnaise total up to 495 calories and 55 grams of fat. Compare that to the mere 59 calories and 3.6 grams of fat in 5 tablespoons of mustard—the mayonnaise/mustard switch offers a 93 percent reduction in fat! Significant reductions in fat content (although usually not as high as 93 percent) occur often in my nutrition work. Rather than take food away from people, I simply replace the poor food choices with healthy alternatives.

"Now I've got a chance!" Connie said as she left my office. Indeed she has, and so does every obese person who follows the same route. However, the food part of Connie's drive for leanness is the blunt end of the stick; the sharp part for her will be exercise, since moving her bulk around is fatiguing, if not downright painful because nature gave her a lighter person's feet. Two months later, she's more vibrant and her body composition is well on its way to normalcy.

Several Other Examples

Niles Borlander. Sales executive Niles Borlander is about ten years older than Connie. He came in before his obesity was as severe as hers. In spite of being a bit past plump, Niles is a very energetic guy who correctly regards food as an important source of energy. But he goes wrong by not responding to the obvious fact that once his nutritional needs are met, eating more food causes more fat to be stored in his body.

In our initial discussion Niles, who works for a computerization consulting firm, told me he had always eaten something "for energy" before a presentation (a good idea if the right food choices are made). Afterward, Niles would celebrate his success at closing the deal—or console himself for failing to do so—by going to the nearest restaurant and putting away a calorically dense dessert. For a few years (as his face puffed up and his stomach pushed out) things seemed to be going extremely well for Niles. In a 40-person sales force, he regularly brought in 5 percent of the company's business—double the average performance.

But things began to change when a new sales manager, a fitness enthusiast, took over and began giving the choice opportunities to new salespeople. Niles felt slighted, and his sales suffered. When he complained, he was told, "We need more lean, mean, and hungry people out beating the bushes for us." When Niles came to see me, he felt he had to lose weight or change jobs, and he didn't want to start over somewhere else.

I presented the Anti-Diet philosophy and exercise schedule and assured Niles it would turn him into a lean, mean sales machine in six to eight months—if he stayed on it. Niles was enthusiastic about everything except how long it would take and wondered if he would be given so much time to lose weight. I urged Niles to talk frankly with his new boss, discuss his new appreciation of the importance of fitness in sustaining production, outline the steps he was taking, and ask for suggestions and advice on his health-rebuilding plans.

Two months later, Niles called back and said his fitness enthusiast boss had been delighted to discuss fitness and diet with him. He was a bit ahead of schedule on waist reduction. Niles said both his sales production and his enjoyment of life were "way up." "Fitness pays off big—that's the bottom line," he told me.

Dolores Caravelle. Dolores, a bright, fast-talking woman about 40 years old, is the director of product development at a cosmetics manufacturer. Dolores felt she was "a little hippy."

Dolores is ambitious. In her highly image-conscious field, she believes carrying extra pounds around her middle is detrimental to her career. She mentioned something equally important to her: At the end of the day she was always exhausted, and even in the mornings she lacked the energy she had possessed before gaining her last 20 pounds.

When she came in, Dolores told me that she had failed to derive any lasting benefit from several spot-reducing programs. She was ready to take a realistic approach to her problem.

I told Dolores that our bodies have a thin layer of fat all over, but in some places it's somewhat thicker. So, as she reduces, she will lose a little all over, and her hips might always be a little bigger, no matter what she does. Then I tailored a program to her needs and interests.

She embarked on a permanent lifestyle change to the Anti-Diet program. When I saw her again eight months later, the change in her face was remarkable. Good nutrition combined with aerobic exercise had done its reliable work; she was slimmer all over, looked terrific, and said she felt great. And she no longer referred to herself as being "hippy."

Oprah Winfrey. When Oprah Winfrey started her spectacularly successful drive to reduce, she was in about the same range of obesity as Connie had been. I admire Oprah's courage and confidence to reduce while millions watched. Oprah ate wisely and—under close supervision—worked out twice a day to burn fat and increase fitness. Within months she entered her first marathon and reached the finish line in respectable time. An astonishing, almost unbelievable, feat.

Oprah, Connie, Niles, and Dolores have all proven that with determination and knowledge, plumpness or even obesity can be beaten. You can find the knowledge and strategies in this book; the determination you must find in your heart.

Only You Can Make the Change

During a recent speaking engagement in front of over 250 people, I asked how many people were aware of the importance of nutrition in their daily performance. Everyone in the room raised his or her hand, indicating to me that their awareness was high. Then, I asked the question, "How many are committed to good nutrition in your lives?" Only about ten percent of the audience raised their hands. Commitment was greatly different from awareness.

I believe the media attention to nutrition in the 1980s made us all aware of nutrition and its importance. However, commitment is always difficult, and good nutrition has always been one of the toughest things to commit to and stay focused on.

Making and Keeping a Commitment to Change

As with everything worthwhile in life, making and keeping a commitment to the Anti-Diet takes some effort and planning. Few skills are more valuable. Learning how to do this opens unlimited possibilities.

If you proceed with alert determination, you will succeed. I've broken the process down into nine steps:

1. Think through why you want to make the change, and what benefits will come to you as a result. At this stage, don't consider the difficulties or the process. Think only of the result. Most wishes to change die right here because you tend to focus too soon on the pain of change, on what you might have to give up, on what new thing you might have to do. Get a clear mental picture of what you want to accomplish, and of who and what you want to be.

2. Concentrate on what you want to achieve and the rewards it will bring you. Face up to what you might need to cut back, make the necessary decisions, and refuse to allow the fear of cutbacks to keep you mired in a rut.

3. Give yourself a reality check. A major source of failure is to set impossible goals. Difficult goals that make you stretch to achieve them are great; impossible ones are a time bomb.

4. Simplify your main goal into a single, measurable result that excites you, and write it down. You should be able to state it in a single, short sentence. Be specific. Your goal should be something like, "I'm going to be a district manager in this company, so I can afford to move my family into our dream home."

5. Break your main goal into pieces you can work on. To reach the highest velocity in your career you must function at your top potential. That means putting everything in this book to work for you. If you have settled on a goal that inspires you, you will want to increase your stamina and reach your top level of alertness and cognitive ability. So you'll set up schedules to bring your physical self up to speed by eating, sleeping, and exercising right.

6. Decide how you'll make time and energy available for learning and doing the things your new plans require. Review all your activities. Inevitably, some old activities will have to be cut back or eliminated.

7. Take action to prevent burnout on your improvement plans. Make sure you've allowed enough time and energy to meet your needs for recreation and relaxation. Are you asking too much, too soon, of yourself? If so, look for things you don't have to do.

8. Set up checkpoints to monitor your progress. Frequently revise your plan, and even your goals, to take advantage of new developments.

9. Persist. Expect to meet disappointments and setbacks. Avoid carving your success timetable in stone. The most successful people all know that persistence is the essence of accomplishment.

Chapter 11

VITAMINS, MINERALS, AND OTHER ADDITIVES FOR YOUR REFUELING STOPS

"Taking huge daily doses of vitamins and minerals over and above the amounts required to fulfill your body's needs, <u>won't</u> power your brain or help you manage your moods."
—Judith J. Wurtman, Ph.D.

Outside the pill industry, there's virtual agreement among dietitians and nutrition researchers that it's far better to get your vitamins and minerals from food rather than from pills. This conviction is based on findings that more vitamins and minerals are absorbed when they're obtained from food than when they come from pills. It's unwise to rely on pills for vitamins and minerals instead of eating a nutritiously dense diet.

Vitamins and minerals are called micronutrients, meaning you don't require a lot of them each day, but you definitely need some of them. They are essential for many bodily functions and processes. Without vitamin C, your body would have trouble fighting infection; without vitamin E, your circulatory system would falter; without calcium, your bones would become brittle; without iron, your body could not produce life-essential hemoglobin in the blood. No matter how well you think you eat, you must be sure (as Mom always said) that you're getting your vitamins and minerals.

How Well Do You Eat?

This is a typical daily diet of a person who thinks she eats well. She is 38 years old, 5 feet 5 inches tall, weighs 125 pounds, and is moderately active.

Breakfast:
1 cup Shredded Wheat cereal with 1/2 cup low-fat milk;
banana; 2 cups of coffee.
Lunch:
Turkey sandwich on whole wheat; salad with low-calorie
dressing; iced tea.
Dinner:
Baked chicken breast (no skin); baked potato; salad with
low-calorie dressing; frozen yogurt.
Here's the analysis of her diet for that day, showing the
nutrients she consumed as a percent of her Recommended
Daily Allowance:

Item	Quantity	%RDA
Total Calories	1045	50
*Carbohydrates	153 g	51
Fiber	16.5 g	79
Calcium	294 mg	37
Iron	7.66 mg	51
Zinc	6.01 mg	50

*53.5 g (35 percent) of her total carbohydrates were from simple sugar.

The following nutrients were also less than 100 percent of
her RDA: Vitamins A, B_1, B_2, D, E, Pantothenic Acid, and
minerals copper and sodium.
    She is eating her way into several vitamin and mineral defi-
ciencies. Her low intakes of calcium and iron are particularly
dangerous. She needs to add foods rich in calcium and iron,
consume seven servings a day of fresh fruits and vegetables,
and take a vitamin and mineral supplement.

What's the Latest on Vitamin and Mineral Supplements?

    Everyone believes that "if you eat a high-calorie, well-bal-
anced diet, you do not need a vitamin/mineral supplement." In
theory, that's the honest truth, but in practice it's almost impossible to achieve, especially if you travel a lot. I know because I
travel extensively, and I try to eat well.
    For 30 days I monitored my dietary intake, recording

everything that went into my stomach. After the 30 days, I evaluated each day and found this: I had gained weight (trying to eat everything I needed), and I had a shortage in some vitamins and minerals.

Interestingly, I recently read that 85 percent of all registered dietitians take a vitamin/mineral supplement. After studying this further, I surmised that it's virtually impossible to eat all fresh foods (avoiding processed foods) and get all your basic nutrients.

So, can you go a day or two without getting exactly "what the doctor ordered" in terms of vitamins and minerals without incurring problems? The answer is, "Sure," but I don't recommend it.

It's true that the body adapts. For example, let's say you haven't had any vitamin C for a few days and that you eat an orange. Your body says, "Hey, I don't get this vitamin C too often, so I've got to get as much as I can!" Does that work in practice? Don't bet your health on it because the jury is still out!

I recommend you take a multivitamin, multimineral supplement each day. There are many excellent brands that are all satisfactory: Anti-Diet Vitamin/Mineral Supplements*, Theragram, GNC, Interior Design Nutritionals, Shaklee, Rexall, and so forth. Look at it this way: It's an inexpensive insurance policy

Many people will tell you that it's much better to consume something that is naturally grown, that comes from real living things. On the surface that seems logical, but it's not true. Research has established that your body doesn't know the difference between an organic vitamin or an inorganic one. It absorbs and assimilates synthetics to the same extent that it utilizes vitamins from natural sources.

Don't Overdo It.

We know deficiencies in folic acid and vitamin B_{12} can impair mental and emotional well-being, but there's no evidence that high doses of them help people think faster or feel better. The whole idea of overdosing to extend the benefits of some nutrient or other may spring from an unconscious analogy to

*Please contact LGE Sport Scinece at 1-800-543-7764 for information about Anti-Diet Vitamin/Mineral Supplements and other products.

stepping on the gas. In reality, a better analogy is to filling up the gas tank: Once it's full, your car can't use more gasoline. It's the same with nutrition: Once you've filled up your daily requirement of all the things you need, consuming more of them can't make you go faster.

Vitamins A, E, D, and K are the four fat-soluble vitamins. If you take megadoses of these, you can create a toxic problem because your body stores these vitamins. Vitamin C and the B-complex vitamins are water-soluble, so if you take too much of them, they are flushed away that day.

Don't get carried away, however. If you start taking 5,000 milligrams of vitamin C, you will just urinate it away and increase the possibility of causing kidney stones.

About two-thirds of corporate America takes a vitamin/mineral supplement. I'm convinced it's not as easy to meet the RDAs for all the vitamins and minerals as has often been claimed. So I recommend a supplement, but not mega-doses. Overdosing on vitamins and minerals can't have a therapeutic effect. Vitamins and minerals are not drugs; they are simply substances that your body must have to continue its normal functions. Once you get enough of a vitamin, you don't need more. If it's the kind of vitamin or mineral that the body can store, there's a risk of toxic effects from the overdose. If it's not storable, it will be excreted. Large overdoses of those that can be excreted can also cause problems.

There are two common beliefs associated with vitamins and minerals, and they are both wrong: They will not energize you like Superman or Wonder Woman, nor will they sedate you or relieve all your stress. They are simply catalysts to help your body function—that's all they do. But we do need them, and so I recommend a supplement that has multivitamins and multi-minerals including antioxidants, which help combat the free radicals in your system.

What Is All This Hype About Antioxidants?

In the normal workings of your metabolism, unstable substances called *free radicals* are created in your body. The development of the radicals is compounded as you are exposed to various forms of adverse stimulation. Factors such as smoking (or even exposure to secondary smoke), smog, radiation, ozone exposure, and even physical exercise enhance free radical development. A free radical has a normal proton nucleus that is supposed to have a pair of electrons orbiting around it, but actually it is missing one electron. This unstable molecule is very dangerous to your system. As soon as it's released among the cells in your body, it aggressively tries to attract an electron from a healthy and stable molecule. Once it grabs an electron, it becomes stable and is no longer a free radical. But the molecule it stole the electron from is now a free radical—and it goes on the rampage to find another electron to become stabilized. The process is ongoing, becoming a chain reaction. Research today estimtates that each of your body molecules gets about 100,000 hits a day from free radicals trying to steal electrons. It is this constant bombardment of cells that causes potential carcinogenic situations to develop in your body.

The terms "antioxidants" and "free radicals" sound like marketing gimmicks dreamed up on Madison Avenue to sell pills. But free radicals are real, and we need antioxidants to combat them.

Free radicals occur in our basic metabolism. The higher the metabolism, the more free radicals are created. Other toxins such as pollution cause free radicals. We either take free radicals in or produce them in the body. Oxidizing free radicals causes them to attack the cells of the body. Scientists theorize that free radicals are partially, and possibly wholly, responsible for the results of aging, such as the changes that take place in cells and the development of heart disease.

We can minimize the impact of free radicals with antioxidants. Antioxidants prevent the premature oxidation of free radicals, which means they can't go in and cause problems.

Research suggests that low-density lipoprotein (LDL) cholesterol—the kind that clogs arteries—only sticks to artery walls when it has been chemically damaged or oxidized by free radicals. It appears that a diet high in olive, canola, or peanut oil and that excludes butter and mayonnaise reduces the tendency of LDL to oxidize. Substituting olive oil, canola oil, or peanut oil for butter and mayonnaise will go far toward keeping your arteries from clogging up. Monounsaturated fats also tend to keep the blood thinner, so it's less likely to block a coronary artery and set off a heart attack.

What Can You Do?

Nutritional science has discovered a way over the last several years to provide your body with substances that have extra electrons. That way, bodily cells wouldn't be continually bombarding one another to regain their stability.

Four substances in nature have been identified to carry out this important mission. *Antioxidants,* as they are called, include the beta carotene in vitamin A, vitamin C, and vitamin E, along with the mineral selenium. Each has the potential to add stability to your body's internal environment. But please don't start buying megadoses of these substances.

You can get most of your antioxidants from natural sources. For example, carrots are loaded with vitamin A, oranges with vitamin C, green leafy vegetables with vitamin E, and Brazil nuts with selenium. However, if that's not the route you choose to take and you prefer taking supplements, here's what I recommend:

Vitamin A: 10,000 I.U.s (I.U. = International Unit)
Vitamin C: 250 to 500 mg
Vitamin E: 200 to 400 I.U.s
Selenium: 70 mcg for adult men and
                  55 mcg for adult women

For a more accurate and individualized selenium recommendation, multiply your weight in pounds by .4 to get your daily allotment of this important antioxidant.

High doses of selenium are toxic. Serious problems can result from overdosing: loss of hair and diarrhea being only two. It's virtually impossible to overdose on selenium from food, but it's a real danger when taking supplements.

Table of Vitamins, Functions, and Sources

Space does not permit a compete listing of every function of each vitamin—only the most important or best known are given here:

A
Functions: Important to good vision and reproduction. Deficiencies cause some kinds of impotence. Helps develop healthy skin, hair, and bones.
Sources: Broccoli, carrots, dark green leafy or yellow-orange-red vegetables; mango and papaya.

B_1 *(Thiamine)*
Functions: Promotes the release of energy from carbohydrates and helps to synthesize nerve-regulating substances.
Sources: Whole-wheat cereals, nuts, legumes, liver, oysters, pork, sunflower seeds, and milk.

B_2 *(Riboflavin)*
Functions: Needed to release stored energy for use and is required for the function of vitamins B_6 (pyrodoxine) and B_3 (niacin). Essential to the metabolism of carbohydrates, fats, and protein. Necessary for building and maintaining body tissues and for many other functions.
Sources: Whole grains, pasta, mushrooms, milk, green vegetables, almonds, oysters, and cottage cheese.

B_3 *(Niacin)*
Functions: Energy production within the body. Necessary for healthy skin.
Sources: Legumes, beans, poultry, peanuts, peas, meat, fish, almonds, and sunflower seeds.

B_6 *(Pyrodoxine)*
Functions: Necessary for the metabolism of protein. Needs increase when more protein is eaten. Also required for the functioning of the nervous system.
Sources: Fish, meat, eggs, kidneys, milk, and oysters.

C
Functions: Besides neutralizing free radicals as an antioxidant, vitamin C plays a major role in fighting infections. It also helps maintain bones, teeth, and blood vessels.
Sources: Fruits, strawberries, tomatoes, potatoes, melons, broccoli, and cauliflower.

D
Functions: Helps the body absorb calcium.
Sources: Exposure to strong sunlight; fish, eggs, and milk.

E
Functions: One of the four antioxidants, vitamin E helps sweep up free radicals. Also helps form red blood cells, muscles, and other tissues.
Sources: Wheat bread, green leafy vegetables, whole-grain cereal, liver, peanuts, and oatmeal.

K
Functions: Helps process substances that are important in blood clotting.
Sources: Leafy green vegetables, cabbage, and soybean oil.

Table of Minerals, Functions, and Sources

Boron
Functions: Essential to calcium metabolism. Works with other minerals to prevent calcium loss.
Sources: Fruits and vegetables, especially apples, pears, broccoli, and carrots.

Calcium
Functions: Necessary to the maintenance of bones, teeth, the transmission of nerve impulses, and muscle contraction.
Sources: Milk, cheese, peas, and dark green leafy vegetables.

Chromium
Functions: Important in carbohydrate metabolism. Aids in the manufacture of red blood cells, the absorption and transfer of iron, and healing.
Sources: Legumes, seafood, nuts, seeds, whole grains, and vegetables.

Iodine
Functions: Necessary for normal cell metabolism and for the prevention of goiters.
Sources: Primarily iodized salt, but widely found in the food supply, especially in seafood and dairy products.

Iron
Functions: Essential to the development of hemoglobin.
Sources: Lean meats, fish, poultry, nuts, seeds, whole grains, green leafy vegetables.

Magnesium
Functions: Necessary for many basic metabolic processes. Helps to hold calcium in tooth enamel and relaxes muscles after contraction. Helps in the conduction of nerve impulses and in the functions of several enzymes.
Sources: Green vegetables, nuts, seeds, legumes, chocolate, and poultry.

Manganese
Functions: Activates some enzymes needed to utilize vitamin B1 (thiamine) and vitamin C. Plays a role in bone development.
Sources: Whole grains, nuts, vegetables, fruit, instant coffee, tea, and cocoa powder.

Phosphorus
Functions: Required for energy production, it also helps form bones, teeth, cell membranes, and genetic material.
Sources: Poultry, fish, meats, milk, eggs, grains, and legumes.

Potassium
Functions: Needed for muscle contraction, nerve impulses, and the proper action of the heart and kidneys. Helps regulate blood pressure and the water balance in cells.
Sources: Most foods, particularly oranges and orange juice, bananas, potatoes with skin, whole grains, and most meat and dairy products.

Selenium
Functions: An antioxidant that helps regulate free radicals, selenium is essential to the immune response and the functioning of the heart muscle.
Sources: Meats, seafood, eggs, whole grains, legumes, and Brazil nuts.

Sodium *(Salt)*
Functions: Regulation of the body's fluid balance, generation of nerve impulses, and the metabolism of carbohydrates and protein.
Sources: Processed foods and table salt.

Zinc
Functions: Metabolism of protein, carbohydrates, fats, and
alcohol. Necessary for many enzyme functions, the synthesis
of proteins, tissue growth, and the healing of wounds.
Sources: Seafood, meat, liver, eggs, milk, and whole-wheat
bread.

APPENDIX

If you would like LGE Sport Science to do your nutrition profile, please send $100 by check, money order, or credit card number (Visa/MC) and follow these instructions:

1. Mail or fax your name, address and phone number, age, height, current weight, gender (if female, please note if you're pregnant or lactating), and your activity level. The definition of activity level is:

Sedentary: No activity to little activity: less than 1 hour each week.

Lightly active: 1 to 2 hours of activity each week.

Moderately active: At least 3 hours of exercise and physical activity weekly.

Very active: On your feet a lot, plus 6 to 9 hours of exercise per week.

Extremely active: At least 2 to 3 hours of *strenuous* activity each day.

2. Now, record everything you eat and drink for two full days. Don't just report that you had a salad or sandwich. Please detail what composed the salad or sandwich. *(Salad example:* 2 cups of iceberg lettuce, 2 tablespoons of grated carrots, 2 tablespoons of chopped tomatoes, 2 cucumber slices with 2 tablespoons of fat-free ranch dressing. *Sandwich example*: two slices of whole-wheat bread, 2 ounces of sliced turkey breast, 1 tablespoon of mustard.) Here is an example for one day:

Jeanne Doe: Female, age, 42; height, 5 feet 4 inches; weight, 129 pounds; activity level, moderately active.

Breakfast: 1 cup oatmeal with 1 cup skim milk; 1 cup chopped melon; 2 cups of coffee.

Snack: 1 banana

Lunch: 3 cups of lettuce, 2 ounces sliced turkey, 1 ounce sliced ham, 1 cup chopped tomatoes, 2 tablespoons of grated carrots, 3 cucumber slices, 4 tablespoons of oil and vinegar dressing, 1 cup vegetarian vegetable soup, 8 ounces iced tea without sugar.

Snack: 1 apple

Dinner: 6 ounces broiled swordfish, 1 baked potato with skin, 1 cup mixed vegetables, 1 cup mixed fruit.

Send your information to:

LGE Sport Science, Inc.
9757 Lake Nona Road
Orlando, FL 32827
1-800-543-7764 (1-800-LGE-PROG)
Fax (407) 438-6667

My Personal Challenge to You

You've heard that life is a journey—a long distance race, not a sprint. And that journey is to be enjoyed day by day, hour by hour, and minute by minute. The same idea can be applied to proper nutrition.

Life should be fun—so should eating.

Life prepares us for challenges—so does nutrition.

Success depends on how you live your life—and how you live your life can be enhanced by good nutrition.

Life is demanding—nutrition helps us respond to those demands.

The body is adaptable—train yourself to enjoy eating well.

I grew up in the Midwest. Popular thinking in my childhood was that you got energy from fat. And fatten up I did right after college. I only got a handle on good nutrition and exercise in my late 20s. I had to change my habits, and you can too.

Now, I eat what I want, when I want it. Your joyful journey through life depends on the decision you will now make. I wish you the best on your journey.

—Jack Groppel

BIBLIOGRAPHY—NUTRITION

Acworth, I.N.; During, M.J.; and Wurtman, R.J. "Tyrosine: Effects of Catecholamine Release." *Brain Research Bulletin* 21 (1988). 3:474-77.

Anderson, I. and Cowen, P. "Neuroendocrine Responses to L-Tryptophan as Index of Brain Serotonin Function: Effect of Weight Loss." *Advances in Experimental Medicine and Biology* (1991). 294:245.

Asheychik, R.; Jackson, T.; Baker, H.; Ferraro, R.; Ashton, T.; and Kilgore, J. "The Efficacy of L-Tryptophan in the Reduction of Sleep Disturbance and Depressive State in Alcoholic Patients." *Journal of Studies on Alcohol* 50 (1989). 5:525.

Astrup, A., et al. "Caffeine: A Double-Blind, Placebo-Controlled Study of Its Thermogenic, Metabolic, and Cardiovascular Effects on Healthy Volunteers." *American Journal of Clinical Nutrition* (1990). 52:759.

Baer, R.A. "Effects of Caffeine on Classroom Behavior, Sustained Attention, and a Memory Task in Preschool Children." *Journal of Applied Behavior Analysis* 20 (1987). 3:225.

Benzi, G.; Marzatico, F.; Pastoris, O.; and Villa, R.F. "Relationship Between Aging, Drug Treatment, and the Cerebral Enzymatic Antioxidant System." *Experimental Gerontology* 24 (1989). 2:137.

Bergstrom, J. "Diet, Muscle Glycogen, and Physical Performance." *Acta Physiologica Scandanavia* (1967). 71:40.

Bes, A.; Dupui, P.; Guell, A.; Bessoles, G.; and Geraud, G. "Pharmacological Exploration of Dopamine Hypersensitivity in Migraine Patients." *International Journal of Clinical Pharmacology Research* 6 (1986). 3:1989.

Bindoli, A.; Rigobello, M.P.; and Deble, D.J. "Biochemical and Toxicological Properties of the Oxidation Products of Catecholamines." *Free Radical Biology & Medicine* (1992). 13:391.

Blumberg, Jeffrey G. "Dietary Antioxidants and Aging." *Contemporary Nutrition* 17 (1992). 3:1.

Bowden, Jonathan. "Fat Facts and Fallacies." *Idea Personal Trainer* (March/April 1995): 44.

Bucci, L.; Hickson J.F.; Wolinsky, I.; et al. "Ornithine Supplementation and Insulin Release in Bodybuilders." *International Journal of Sports Nutrition* (1992). 2:287.

Byers, Tim and Perry, Geraldine. "Dietary Carotenes, Vitamin C, and Vitamin E as Protective Antioxidants in Human Cancers." *Annual Review of Nutrition* (1992). 12:139-59.

Byers, Tim, et al., "New Directions: The Diet-Cancer Link." *Patient Care* (November 30, 1990): 34ff.

Contijoch, A.M.; Johnson, A.L.; and Advis, J.P. "Norepinephrine-Stimulated in Vitro Release of Lutenizing Hormone-Releasing Hormone (LHRH) from Median Eminence Tissue Facilitated by Inhibition of LHRH-Degrading Activity in Hens." *Biology of Reproduction* 42 (1990). 2:222.

Costill, D.; Coyle, E.; and Dalsky, G. "Effect of Plasma FFA and Insulin on Muscle Glycogen Usage During Exercise." *Journal of Applied Physiology* (1977). 42:695.

Daly, P.A.; Krieger, D.R.; Dulloo, A.G.; et al. "Ephedrine, Caffeine, and Aspirin: Safety and Efficacy for Treatment of Human Obesity." *International Journal of Obesity* 17 (1993). Supplement 1: S73-78.

Daly, P.A. and Landsberg, L. "Hypertension in Obesity and NIDDM: Role of Insulin and Sympathetic Nervous System." *Diabetes Care* (1991). 14:240-248.

D'Andrea, G.; Cananzi, A.R.; Grigoletto, F.; et al. "The Effect of Dopamine Receptor Agonists on Prolactin Secretion in Childhood Migraine." *Headache* 28 (1988). 5:354.

Dawson-Hughes, Bess. "Nutrition, Exercise, and Lifestyle Factors that Affect Bone Health," in Frank Kotsonis and Maureen Mackey, eds., *Nutrition in the 90s* (New York: Marcel Dekker, 1994). 2:99-116.

Dietz, Jane M., et al. "Effects of Thermal Processing Upon Vitamins and Proteins in Foods." *Nutrition Today* (July/August 1989): 6-14.

Domel, S.B.; Baranowski, T.; Leonard, S.B.; Litaker, M.S.; Baranowski, J.; Mullis, R.; Byers, T.; Strong, W.B.; Treiber, F.; and Levy, M. "Defining the Year 2000 Fruit and Vegetable Goal." *Journal of the American College of Nutrition* 12 (December 1993) 6:669.

Dulloo, A. and Miller, D.S. "Ephedrine, Caffeine, and Aspirin: Over-the-Counter Drugs that Interact to Stimulate Thermogenesis in the Obese." *Nutrition* (1989). 5:7.

Elmadfa, I.; Both B.N.; Sierakowski, B.; and Steinhagen, T.E. "Significance of Vitamin E in Aging." *Journal of Gerontology* 19 (1986). 3:206.

Feldman, J.M.; Lee, E.M.; and Castleberry, C.A. "Catecholamine and Serotonin Content of Foods: Effects on Urinary Excretion of Homovanilic and 5-Hydroxyindoleacetic Acid." *Journal of the American Dietetic Association* 87 (August 1987). 8:1031-35.

Fernstrom, J.D. "Tryptophan, Serotonin, and Carbohydrate Appetite: Will the Real Carbohydrate Craver Please Stand Up!" *Journal of Nutrition* (April 1988). 118:1417-19.

Flynn, M.A.; Nolph, G.B.; and Krause, G. "Comparison of Body Composition by Total Body Potassium and Infrared Interactance." *Journal of the American College of Nutrition* 14 (December 1995). 6:652.

George, C.F.; Millar, T.W.; Hanly, P.J.; and Kryger, M.H. "The Effects of L-Tryptophan on Daytime Sleep Latency in Normals: Correlation with Blood Levels. *Sleep* 12 (1989). 4:345.

Greenburg, S. and Frishman, W.H. "Co-Enzyme Q_{10}: A New drug for Cardiovascular Disease." *Journal of Clinical Pharmacology* 30 (1990). 7:596.

Haeckel, R.; Colic, D.; Binder, L.; and Ollerich, M. "Stimulation of Glucose Metabolism in Human Blood Cells by Inhibitors of Carnitine-Dependent Fatty Acid Transport." *Journal of Clinical Chemistry and Clinical Biochemistry* 28 (1990) 5:329.

Harris, William S. "The Prevention of Atherosclerosis with Antioxidants." *Clinical Cardiology* (1992). 15:636-40.

Hull, E.M.; Bazzett, T.J.; Warner, R.K.; Eaton, R.C.; and Thompson, J.T. "Dopamine Receptors in the Entral Tegmental Area Modulate Male Sexual Behavior in Rats." *Brain Research* 512 (1990). 1:1.

Idzikowski, C. and Oswald, I. "Interference with Human Memory by an Antibiotic." *Psychopharmacology* 79 (1983). 2:2.

Ikonian, T. "Mood Food." *Men's Fitness* (August 1993): 33-35.

Ivy, J. "Muscle Glycogen Synthesis After Exercise and Effect of Time on Carbohydrate Ingestion." *Journal of Applied Physiology* (1988). 64:1480-85.

Jaedig, S. and Henningsen, N.C. "Increased Metabolic Rate in Obese Women After Ingestion of Potassium, Magnesium, and Phosphate-Enriched Orange Juice or Injection of Ephedrine." *International Journal of Obesity* 15 (1991). 6:426.

Jenkins, David. "Health Benefits of Complex Carbohydrates and Fiber," in Frank Kotsonis and Maureen Mackey, eds. *Nutrition in the 90s* (New York: Marcel Dekker, 1994). 2:15-24.

Jenkins, R.R., et al. "Introduction: Oxidant Stress, Aging, and Exercise." *Medicine & Science in Sports & Exercise* 25 (1993). 2:210-12.

Katts, G.R., et al. "The Short-Term Therapeutic Efficacy of Treating Obesity with a Plan of Improved Nutrition and Moderate Caloric Restriction." *Current Therapeutic Research* (1992). 51:261-72.

Kelly, S.J. and Franklin, K.B. "An Increase in Tryptophan in Brain May Be a General Mechanism for the Effect of Stress on Sensitivity to Pain." *Neuropharmacology* 24 (1985). 11:1019.

Kostas, Georgia G. "Fast Food Eating." *Idea Personal Trainer* (January 1995): 40.

Kurtzam, Felice D. "Stress Eating." *Idea Personal Trainer* (June 1995): 40.

Laymayer, Ruth. "Holiday Eating." *Idea Personal Trainer* (November/December 1995): 40.

Lennon, D.L.; Shrago, E.R.; Madden, M.; Nagle, F.J.; and Hanson, P. "Dietary Carnitine Intake Related to Skeletal Muscle and Plasma Carnitine Concentrations in Adult Men and Women." *American Journal of Clinical Nutrition* 43 (1986). 2:324.

Levitsky, David. "Imprecise of Food Intake on Low-Fat Diets," in Frank Kotsonis and Maureen Mackey, eds. *Nutrition in the 90s*, (New York: Marcel Dekker, 1994). 2:45-60.

Loke, W.H. "Effects of Caffeine on Mood and Memory." *Physiology & Behavior* 44 (1988). 3:367.

Mackey, M. and Hill, Betsy P. "Health Claims Regulations and New Food Concepts," in Frank Kotsonis and Maureen Mackey, eds. *Nutrition in the 90s* (New York: Marcel Dekker, 1994). 2:143-64.

Maher, T.J. and Wurtman, R.J. "Possible Neurologic Effects of Aspartame, a Widely Used Food Additive." *Environmental Health Perspective* (1987). 75:53.

Mann, J. "Nutrition Options When Reducing Saturated Fat Intake." *Journal of the American College of Nutrition* 11 (June 1992). Supplement:82S.

Mathura, C.B.; Singh, H.H.; Tizabi, Y.; Hughes, J.E.; and Flesher, S.A. "Effects of Chronic Tryptophan Loading on Serotonin (5-HT) Levels in Neonatal Rat Brain." *Journal of the American Medical Association* 78 (1986). 7:645.

Maurizi, C.P. "The Therapeutic Potential for Tryptophan and Melatonin: Possible Roles in Depression, Sleep, Alzheimer's Disease and Abnormal Aging." *Medical Hypotheses* 66 (1990). 4:504.

Milner, I. "Health-Food Industry Sells Supplements, Not Science." *Environmental Nutrition* (January 1990). 13:1-3.

"Mother Knows Best," from a study in *Journal of the American Medical Association* [on fruit and vegetable intake] in "What's New." *Idea Personal Trainer* (June 1995): 7.

Mueller, W.H. and Wohleb, J.C. "Anatomical Distribution of Subcutaneous Fat and Its Description by Multivariate Methods: How Valid Are Principal Components?" *American Journal of Physical Anthropology* (1981). 54:25-35.

"No News Is Good News." *Science* (1992). 258:1862.

Pagan, A. and Bonanome, A. "Monosaturated Fatty Acids in Human Nutrition." *Journal of the American College of Nutrition* 11 (June 1992). Supplement:79S.

Price, W.A.; Zimmer, B.; and Kucas, P. "Serotonin Syndrome: A Case Report." *Journal of Clinical Pharmacology* 26 (1986). 1:77.

"Revised Weight Guidelines," in "What's New." *Idea Personal Trainer* (November/December 1995): 7.

Ribaya-Mercado, J.D.; Ordovas, J.M.; Russell. "Effect of ß-Carotene Supplementation on the Concentrations and Distribution of Carotenoids, Vitamin E, Vitamin A, and Cholesterol in Plasma Lipoprotein and Nonlipoprotein Fractions of Healthy Older Women." *Journal of the American College of Nutrition* 14 (December 1995). 6:604.

Rodriguez, Nancy. "Food or Fiction?" *Idea Personal Trainer* (September 1995): 26.

Rose, David P. "Dietary Fat, Fiber, and Cancer," in Frank Kotsonis and Maureen Mackey, eds. *Nutrition in the 90s* (New York: Marcel Dekker, 1994). 2:1-14.

Schneider, H.D. "[Treatment of Sleep Disorders with L-Tryptophan: Uses of Interval Therapy in Severe Insomnia and Hypnotic Dependence]" *Fortschritte der Medizin* 105 (1987). 6:113.

Silverstone, T. "Mood and Food: A Psychopharmacological Enquiry." *Annals New York Academy of Sciences* (1987). 499:264-68.

Sindrup, S.H.; Gram, L.F.; Brosen, K.; Eshoj, O.; and Mogensen, E.F. "The Selective Serotonin Reuptake Inhibitor Paroxetine Is Effective in the Treatment of Diabetic Neuropathy Symptoms." *Pain* 42 (1990). 2:135.

Skolnik, Heidi and Wein, Debra. "Nutrition in Question." *Idea Personal Trainer* (March/April 1995): 11.

Slattery, M.L.; Jacobs, D.R.; Dyer, A.; Benson, J.; Hilner, J.E.; and Caan, B.J. "Dietary Antioxidants and Plasma Lipids: The Cardia Study." *Journal of the American College of Nutrition* 14 (December 1995). 6:635.

Smith, F.L.; Yu, D.S.; Smith, D.G.; Leccese, A.P.; and Lyness, W.H. "Dietary Tryptophan Supplements Attenuate Amphetamine Self-Administration in the Rat." *Pharmacology, Biochemistry & Behavior* 25 (1986). 4:849.

Sommi, R.W.; Crimson, M.L.; Bowden, C.L.; et al. "Fluoxetine: A Serotonin-Specific, Second-Generation Antidepressant." *Pharmacotherapy* 9 (1987). 5:529.

Sottovia, Carla. "How Accurate Is My Body Fat Assessment?" *Idea Personal Trainer* (May 1995): 18.

"Spotlight on Soy," from a study in Tufts University Diet and Nutrition Letter [on phytoestrogens and cancer] in "What's New." *Idea Personal Trainer* (September 1995): 12.

Tayarani, I.; Cloez, I.; Clement, M.; and Bourre, J.M. "Antioxidant Enzymes and Related Trace Elements in Aging Brain Capillaries and Choroid Plexus." *Journal of Neurochemistry* 53 (1989). 5:817.

Thomas, John A. "Transgene Technology: Impact on Nutritional Research," in Frank Kotsonis and Maureen Mackey, eds. *Nutrition in the 90s* (New York: Marcel Dekker, 1994). 2:133-42.

U.S. Department of Agriculture and U.S. Department of Health and Human Services. *Nutrition and Your Health: Dietary Guidelines for Americans.* 4th edition. (Washington, DC: U.S. Department of Agriculture, 1995). Home and Garden Bulletin No. 232.

Volger, B.W. "Alternatives in the Treatment of Memory Loss in Patients with Alzheimer's Disease." *Clinical Pharmacy* 10 (1991). 6:227.

Wahlqvist, Mark L. "New Directions in Food-Health Research," in Frank Kotsonis and Maureen Mackey, eds. *Nutrition in the 90s* (New York: Marcel Dekker, 1994). 2:117-32.

Waslien, Carol I., et al. "Micronutrients and Antioxidants in Processed Foods—Analysis of Data from 1987 Food Additives Survey." *Nutrition Today* (July/August 1990): 36ff.

Williams, Roger R. "Diet, Genes, Early Heart Attacks, and High Blood Pressure," in Frank Kotsonis and Maureen Mackey, eds. *Nutrition in the 90s* (New York: Marcel Dekker, 1994). 2:25-44.

Willson, R. "Free Radical Protection: Why Vitamin E—Not Vitamin C, Beta-Carotene or Glutathione?" *Ciba Foundation Symposium* 101 (London: Pitman Publishing, 1983): 19.

Wurtman, J.J. "Neurotransmitter Control of Carbohydrate Consumption." *Annals New York Academy of Sciences* (1985). 443:145-51.

Wurtman, R.J. "Dietary Treatments that Affect Brain Neurotransmitters." *Annals New York Academy of Sciences* (1987). 499:179-90.

Yokogoshi, H. and Nomura, M. "Effect of Amino Acid Supplementation to a Low-Protein Diet on Brain Neurotransmitters and Memory-Learning Ability of Rats." *Physiology & Behavior* 50 (1991). 6:1227.

Young, S.N. "Acute Effects of Meals on Brain Tryptophan and Serotonin in Humans." *Advances in Experimental Medicine & Biology* (1991). 294:417.

Zempleni, J. "Pharmacokinetics of Vitamin B_6 Supplements in Humans." *Journal of the American College of Nutrition* 14 (December 1995). 6:579.

BIBLIOGRAPHY—EXERCISE

American College of Sports Medicine. "Physical Activity, Physical Fitness, and Hypertension." *Medicine & Science in Sports & Exercise* (1993). 25:i-x.

American College of Sports Medicine. "The Recommended Quantity and Quality of Exercise for Developing and Maintaining Fitness in Healthy Adults." *Medicine & Science in Sports & Exercise* (1978). 10:vii-x.

American Heart Association. "Exercise Standards: A Statement for Healthcare Professionals from The American Heart Association." *Circulation* (1995). 91:580-96.

Ali, N.S. and Twibell, R.K. "Health Promotion and Osteoporosis Prevention Among Postmenopausal Women." *Preventive Medicine* (1995). 24:528-34.

Beltz, J.D.; Costill, D.L.; Thomas, R.; Fink, W.J.; and Kirwan, J.P. "Energy Demands of Interval Training for Competitive Swimming." *Journal of Swimming Research* 4 (1988). 3:5-9.

Blair, S.N.; Piserchia, P.V.; Wilbur, C.S.; and Crowder, J.H. "A Public Health Intervention Model for Worksite Health Promotion: Impact on Exercise and Physical Fitness in a Health Promotion Plan After 24 Months." *Journal of the American Medical Association* (1986). 255:921-26.

Borra, S.T; Schwartz, N.E.; Spain, C.G.; and Natchipolsky, M.M. "Food, Physical Activity, and Fun: Inspiring America's Kids to More Healthful Lifestyles." *Journal of the American Dietetic Association* (1995). 7:816-18.

Bouchard, C. and Lortie, G. "Heredity and Endurance Performance." *Sports Medicine* (1984). 1:38-64.

Brodigan, D. "Osteoporosis: The Effect of Exercise Variables." *Melopmene Journal* 11 (1992). 2:16-25.

Broeder, C.E.; Burrhus, K.A.; Svanevik, L.S.; and Wilmore, J.H. "The Effects of Either High Intensity Resistance or Endurance Training on Resting Metabolic Rate." *American Journal of Clinical Nutrition* (1992). 55:802-10.

Burk, C. and Kimiecik, J. "Examining the Relationship Among Locus of Control, Value, and Exercise." *Health Values* (1994). 18:14-23.

Campbell, W.W., et al. "Increased Energy Requirements and Changes in Body Composition with Resistance Training in Older Adults." *American Journal of Clinical Nutrition* (1994). 60:167-75.

DeBusk, R.F., et al. "Training Effects of Long Versus Short Bouts of Exercise." *American Journal of Cardiology* (1990). 65:1010-13.

Duffy, M.E. and MacDonald, E. "Determinants of Functional Health of Older Persons." *Gerontologist* (1990). 30:503-9.

"Exercise Intensity and Body Composition," from a study in *Journal of the American Dietetic Association* in "What's New." *Idea Personal Trainer* (July/August 1995): 5.

Fielding, R.A. "The Role of Progressive Resistance Training in the Preservation of Lean Body Mass in the Elderly." *Journal of the American College of Nutrition* 14 (December 1995). 6:587.

Frost, H; Moffett, J.A.K.; Moser, J.S.; and Fairbank, J.C.T. "Randomised Controlled Trial for Evaluation of Fitness Programme for Patients with Chronic Low Back Pain." *British Medical Journal* (1995). 310:151-54.

Gaspard, G., et al. "Effects of a Seven-Week Aqua Step Training Program on the Aerobic Capacity and Body Composition of College-Aged Women." *Medicine & Science in Sports & Exercise* 27 (1995). 5: abstract 1011.

Horne, T.E. "Predictors of Physical Activity Intentions and Behaviour for Rural Homemakers." *Canadian Journal of Public Health* (1994). 85:132-35.

Houmard, J.A.; Costill, D.L.; Mitchell, J.B.; Park S.H.; and Chenier, T.C. "The Role of Anaerobic Ability in Middle Distance Running Performance." *European Journal of Applied Physiology* (1991). 62:40-43.

King, A.C.; Haskell, W.L.; Young, D.R.; Oka, R.K.; and Stedfanick, M.L. "Long-Term Effects of Varying Intensities and Formats of Physical Activity on Participation Rates, Fitness, and Lipoproteins in Men and Women Aged 50 to 65 Years." *Circulation* (1995). 91:2596-604.

King, A.C.; Taylor, C.B.; Haskell, W.L.; and Debusk, R.F. "Strategies for Increasing Early Adherence to and Long-Term Maintenance of Home-Based Exercise Training in Healthy Middle-Aged Men and Women." *American Journal of Cardiology* (1988). 61:628-32.

Kuczmarski, R.J.; Flegal, K.M.; Campbell, S.M.; and Johnson, C.L. "Increasing Prevalence of Overweight Among U.S. Adults: The National Health and Nutrition Examination Surveys, 1960 to 1991." *Journal of the American Medical Association* (1994). 272:205-7.

Lee, I.; Hsiech, C.; and Paffenbarger, R. "Exercise Intensity and Longevity in Men: The Harvard Alumni Health Study." *Journal of the American Medical Association* 273 (April 1995). 15:1179-84.

McArdle, W.D.; Katch, F.I.; and Katch, V.L. *Exercise Physiology: Energy, Nutrition, and Human Performance.* 3rd edition. (Philadelphia, PA: Lea & Febiger, 1991).

Mikesky, A.E., et al. "Efficacy of a Home-Based Training Program for Older Adults Using Elastic Tubing." *European Journal of Applied Physiology* (1994). 69:316-20.

Pate, R.R.; Pratt, M.; Blair, S.N.; Haskell, W.L.; Macera, C.A.; Bouchard, C.; et al. "Physical Activity and Public Health: A Recommendation from the Centers for Disease Control and Prevention and the American College of Sports Medicine." *Journal of the American Medical Association* (1995). 273:402-407.

Pavlou, K.N.; Stefee, W.P.; Lerman, R.H.; and Burrows, V. "Effects of Dieting and Exercise on Lean Body Mass, Oxygen Uptake, and Strength." *Medicine and Science in Sports and Exercise* (1985). 17:466-471.

President's Council on Physical Fitness. *The Physician's Rx: Exercise* (Washington, DC: President's Council on Physical Fitness and Sports, 1992).

President's Council on Physical Fitness and Sports and Sporting Goods Manufacturers Association. *American Attitudes Toward Physical Activity and Fitness: A National Survey.* (Washington, DC: President's Council on Physical Fitness and Sports, 1993).

Pronk, N.P.; Course S.F.; and Rohack, J. J. "Maximal Exercises and Acute Mood Response in Women." *Physiology and Behavior* (1995). 57:1-4.

Pyka, G., et al. "Muscle Strength and Fiber Adaptions to a Year-Long Resistance Training Program for Elderly Men and Women." *Journal of Gerontology* (1994). 49:M22-27.

Stefanick, M.L. "Exercise and Weight Control." *Exercise and Sport Science Reviews* (1993). 21:363-96.

"Strength Training and Osteoporosis," from a study in the *Journal of the American Medical Association* in "What's New." *Idea Personal Trainer* (February 1995): 9.

Wallick, et al. "Physiological Responses to In-Line Skating Compared to Treadmill Running." *Medicine & Science in Sports & Exercise* 27 (1995). 2:242-48.

Westcott, Wayne. "High-Intensity Strength Training," [research] in "What's New." *Idea Personal Trainer* (September 1995): 9.

Westcott, Wayne. "High-Intensity Strength Training." *Idea Personal Trainer* (October 1995): 40.

Williford, H.N., et al. "Training Responses Associated with Bench Stepping and Running in Women." *Medicine & Science in Sports & Exercise* 27 (June 1995 supplement): abstract 1125.

INDEX

ABOUT THE AUTHOR

Jack Groppel, Ph.D., is an internationally recognized authority on the application of sports science to human performance. As a sports scientist, he is an expert in fitness, nutrition, and bioengineering, and the author or editor of over 250 articles. He is a principal of LGE Sport Science, Inc. in Orlando, Florida (along with Jim Loehr and Pat Etcheberry.)

Groppel is a forthright and dynamic advocate of fitness and nutrition education. He consults regularly with the top athletes of many major sports, as well as with *Fortune* 1000 companies, on all aspects of personal performance. Distinguishing Groppel's work is his application of successful sport science techniques to the physical, mental, and spiritual performance of corporate audiences. He has been a pioneer in the development and employment of training techniques and programs that blend sound nutrition, physical activity, and attitudinal training to achieve better health and improved productivity and creativity, whether in the workplace or on the playing field.

Groppel is a Fellow of the American College of Sports Medicine, a nationally accredited certified nutrition specialist, and a recipient of the International Tennis Hall of Fame's Educational Merit Award. He is also Chairman of the National Sport Science Committee for the U.S. Tennis Association and the National Co-chair for USPTA's Tennis Across America, which works in cooperation with the President's Council on Physical Fitness and Sports to provide instructional clinics to over 150,000 people nationwide. Prior to 1987, Groppel was an associate professor of kinesiology and bioengineering at the University of Illinois.

About LGE Sport Science, Inc.

LGE Sport Science is regarded as the world leader in the development and implementation of specialized physical and attitudinal training programs for athletes and corporate clients striving for increased performance and productivity. The company's Mentally Tough training techniques have aided some of the world's best athletes and corporate administrators achieve higher levels of effectiveness and, in many instances, reach milestones previously perceived as unattainable.

Company clients include Estee Lauder, Merrill Lynch, Motorola, State Farm, Bristol Myers Squibb, American Airlines, GTE, IBM, Motorola, Price Waterhouse, Ford, Union Carbide, and Blue Cross/Blue Shield, as well as tennis players Jim Courier, Monica Seles and Michael Chang, Olympic gymnast Wendy Bruce, Olympic speed-skater Dan Jansen, hockey players Mike Richter (of the New York Rangers) and Eric Lindros (of the Philadelphia Flyers), and Master's champion Nick Faldo.

Groppel and his partners at LGE Sport Science, Inc., are frequently quoted experts in their field. Major features on the company and its principals and programs have appeared in *U.S. News and World Report*, *Shape* magazine, *Elle* magazine, *Success* magazine, *Golf Digest*, and *Men's Health*.

For information, contact:

> LGE Sport Science, Inc.
> 9757 Lake Nona Road
> Orlando, FL 32827
> 1-800-543-7764 (1-800-LGE-PROG)
> Fax (407) 438-6667